Contents

Massage as a therapy from ancient times to today. Massage in other
cultures. Massage and aromatherapy as part of the holistic movement
and as used by nurses, beauty therapists and massage therapists.

Types of workplace. Employment opportunities, employment standards
and current legislation, responsibilities of employers and employees.
Personal hygiene.

The working environment and its effect on clients and therapists: size,
decor, temperature, ventilation, privacy and hygiene. Necessary and
suitable equipment. Types of massage couch and how to select. Suitable
linen and accessories. Massage mediums: indications for use.

Client consultation: aims and necessary components, therapist's
manner, record systems. Contraindications to massage, conditions
requiring special care, conditions requiring medical referral. Data
Protection Act.

Features and functions of the systems of the body. Effects of massage on
the systems. Contraindications to massage related to the systems.
Stress: its effects on the body and management of stress by massage.
Aromatherapy massage and the systems of the body.

Hand exercises, client feedback, therapist's posture. Categories of
massage movements: effleurage and stroking, petrissage, percussion,
vibrations and shaking, friction and frictions. Uses, points of care and
contra-indications of each category of massage technique.

Massage and Aromatherapy

A Practical Approach for NVQ Level 3

Lyn Goldberg

Stanley Thornes (Publishers) Ltd

First published in 1995 by:
Stanley Thornes (Publisher) Ltd
Ellenborough House
Wellington Street
CHELTENHAM
GL50 1YD
United Kingdom

A catalogue record for this book is available from the British Library.

ISBN 0 7487 2081 2

Typeset by P&R Typesetters Ltd, Salisbury
Printed and bound in Great Britain at The Bath Press, Avon

Acknowledgements

I am indebted to the following for their help and advice during the preparation of this book:

Sandra Holtby, Dean of the School of Fashion Promotion at the London College of Fashion, for her support.

Carlton Professional and New Concept for their generosity in supplying photographs of couches.

Karen Butler of The London College of Fashion for her advice on the aromatherapy chapters.

Jacky Conduit of The Wolverhampton School of Physiotherapy for her advice on the physiology chapter.

Sharon Hotchkiss for specialist advice on skin penetration of fragrance chemicals.

The media resources and computer staff at The London College of Fashion, especially Patrick Moran, who unscrambled my discs.

Claire Boulton, librarian at the London College of Fashion, for help in obtaining original papers.

My husband and daughters for their tolerance, patience and, more importantly, their medical and legal expertise.

Study matrix for NVQ units

Unit	CO1			CO2		CO4				EO1			EO2		
Element	1	2	3	1	2	1	2	3	4	1	2	3	1	2	3
Chapter 1	•			•	•	•				•					
2		•		•	•	•	•			•			•		
3	•	•	•				•	•			•	•		•	•
4	•	•	•				•	•	•		•		•	•	
5							•	•							
6							•	•							
7							•	•							
8	•	•	•							•	•	•			
9		•											•	•	•

Key to chapters

1 The massage therapist in the workplace
2 The working environment
3 Consultation
4 Massage and the systems of the body
5 Massage techniques
6 The massage routine
7 Adaptations to the massage routine
8 Essential oils for aromatherapy massage
9 Aromatherapy massage and other uses for essential oils

Key to units and elements

Unit CO1   Assess the client for treatment
Element 1   Conduct oral assessment for treatment
Element 2   Conduct physical examination for treatment
Element 3   Draw conclusions and advise on treatment

Unit CO2   Maintain services and operations to meet quality standards
Element 1   Maintain services and operations
Element 2   Maintain the necessary conditions for an effective and safe work environment

Unit C04   Provide body massage
Element 1   Maintain standards of hygiene and personal appearance
Element 2   Prepare for body massage
Element 3   Apply body massage techniques
Element 4   Evaluate the effectiveness of body massage and provide aftercare

Unit E01   Prepare plan and select and blend oils for aromatherapy massage
Element 1   Maintain standards of hygiene and personal appearance
Element 2   Consult client and prepare plan for aromatherapy massage
Element 3   Select and blend oils for aromatherapy massage

Unit E02   Provide aromatherapy massage
Element 1   Prepare for aromatherapy massage
Element 2   Apply aromatherapy massage
Element 3   Evalute the effectiveness of aromatherapy massage and give aftercare advice

Introduction

In recent years there has been an amazing increase in the use of massage as a therapy. Until fairly recently any mention of massage other than that used in osteopathy or physiotherapy to treat some medical conditions was regarded with deep suspicion. The growth and acceptance of therapies complementary to orthodox medicine has led to massage being much more widely accepted as a treatment for all sorts of stress-related problems. Of course massage in one form or another has been used in this country and in most parts of the world since time immemorial, but only now in Britain is it becoming so widely accepted that many men and women are training and becoming professional massage therapists outside the medical field.

The English word 'massage' is probably derived from the Arabic *mass'h*, meaning to press softly. There can hardly be a culture where rubbing or pressing of some sort has not been part of the healing process in the past and in many of them the tradition continues alongside the practice of modern medicine. Very often aromatic oils and herbal remedies have been used with massage to help the healing process and we see a revival of this today in the practice of aromatherapy.

We must assume that just as man found food by trial and error and by an instinctive recognition of his needs, so in illness he must have found some substances which acted as drugs to help fend off disease. Many ancient peoples possessed a considerable knowledge of such drugs, which was passed down from father to son (or more likely from mother to daughter as it was they who prepared food and therefore knew how to prepare a healing potion). Instinct must also have played a large part in the development of physical treatments as instinctive rubbing of a sore part of the body is found to relieve pain or discomfort. This rubbing, developed into a system, becomes massage.

Records show that massage was practised in China as early as 3000 BC – one of the earliest books containing a list of exercises and massage movements dates from this time. Their techniques concentrated on finding points on the body where pressing and rubbing were most effective. These techniques spread to Japan and have developed into the system known today as Shiatsu.

In many American Indian tribes traditional medicine was based on the idea that disease was the result of objects which had become embedded in the body and that removing them would help alleviate the problem. The medicine men had many methods of appearing to remove these objects and often preceded these magical routines with rubbing movements which themselves were pain relieving. The Navahos held lengthy healing ceremonials which would combine all the elements of 'primitive' medicine, religious prayers and dances, magic items such as sand paintings and sticks, but also more rational treatments such as sweat baths, incense, drugs and massage.

Massage is referred to in ancient Hindu books such as the *Ayur-Veda* (Art of Life) which dates from 1800 BC. In Indian villages today there is usually someone expert in massage who will often combine massage treatments with the use of herbs, spices and aromatic oils.

Various forms of massage were used in the Middle East and there are letters from as early as the 7th century BC from a physician in Assyria giving instructions for treatment of his king by applying herbs and vigorous massage until he perspired.

Other cultures with documented references to massage are found in Indonesia, Australia and Tahiti. Captain Cook is said to have been cured of sciatica when Tahitan women used massage on him.

In Europe there is a long history of the use of massage. In Ancient Greece and Rome it was used to revive soldiers and gladiators and was part of the regular lifestyle of wealthy citizens. Physical fitness was very important to the Ancient Greeks with regular competitive races and gymnastic displays being held. Regular massage was prescribed for the athletes to keep them supple and fit. Homer, in the *Odyssey* refers to massage with nutrition and exercise to promote healing and fitness for his soldiers. Greek women are known to have used gymnastics, dancing and massage as part of their beauty regime. The Greek physician Herodotus in the 5th century BC used herbs and oils with massage and his pupil Hippocrates recognised the efficiency of stroking movements towards the heart long before the circulation of the blood was understood. Hippocrates advised physicians to learn massage as, 'rubbing can bind and loosen, can make flesh and cause parts to waste; hard rubbing binds, soft rubbing loosens; much rubbing causes parts to waste, moderate rubbing makes them grow'.

The Romans probably acquired the practice of massage and baths from the Greeks and practitioners followed the directions of Hippocrates. The Roman system of baths played a large part in the life of wealthy citizens. The baths were taken in four stages; first a gradual warming up, then a much hotter bath leading to profuse sweating, which was followed by cooling down in a tepid bath and then a cold plunge. During each stage slaves rubbed down the bathers often using brushes and bone utensils to scrape the skin.

Galen, a noted Roman physician of the 1st century AD who discovered that the arteries contained blood, recommended massage for treatment of injury and disease with the strokes being varied in direction according to the result required. The techniques mentioned in Roman times include pummelling, pinching and squeezing. Julius Caesar is said to have had himself rubbed and pinched all over each day to help his neuralgia.

There are occasional references to massage as a beauty treatment in the middle ages but not much was heard of it from the medical world until the 1570s when Ambroise Pare, a French surgeon, reported that he used friction movements to reduce swelling before treating dislocations of joints. He is known to have classified movements into gentle, medium and vigorous and is credited with successfully treating Mary Queen of Scots with massage.

Over the next three centuries more was heard of massage, and in 1700, in Prussia, the king's physician Hoffman used it with exercise to treat his aristocratic patients. By 1800, an Oxford surgeon, John Grosvenor, was using friction to ease stiff joints and Mr Balfour of Edinburgh used rubbing, percussion and compression for rheumatism and gout. It was a Swedish physiologist Peter Henry Ling who developed a clear system of massage and exercise in the early 1800s and whose terminology is still used today to describe Swedish-style massage. The terms effleurage, petrissage and vibration were used by him as well as friction, rolling and slapping. By the middle of the 19th century, French, German and Dutch physicians were modernising and changing the old skills of rubbing and adopting Ling's methods.

It was a Dutch physician, Dr Johann Metzger, who established massage as part of medical practice. In 1860 he cured the Danish crown prince of a joint infection and developed his methods to agree with the current knowledge of anatomy and physiology. Holland was the first European country to have a massage organisation and journal and many other Dutch physicians carried on Metzger's work. He had followers in other countries including America, but it was his German followers, especially Professor von Mosengeil, who promoted his theories in Britain. In the British Medical Journal of May 1866 Dr William Murrell published an article on *Massage as a Therapeutic Agent* referring to its use by German doctors and by Dr Graham of the Massachusetts Therapeutic Massage Association. Dr Graham claimed to have developed methods of treatments which were later used by a German calligrapher called Julius Wolff. This was a way of treating writers cramp with massage and exercise which was so successful that his method was widely accepted by British doctors. He is also known to have influenced such famous French physicians as Charcot and Lucas-Champonniere. In 1889 Lucas-Champonniere published his book *Massage and Mobilisation in the Treatment of Fractures*.

By the late 1800s British doctors were advocating that nurses should be trained in massage to be used in the medical field and in 1894 a group of women founded the Society of Trained Masseuses. These women, while having nursing backgrounds, were interested in developing and regulating physical treatments which, as we have seen, has roots going back into ancient history.

In about 1885 there was an article published in a manual called *The Family Physician* which was a warning from doctors to the general public about massage as a career for young women. This said that there was no demand for people to train as masseuses and that the only people likely to make an income from it are, 'the not over scrupulous people who give lessons and persuade unwary women that it is lucrative employment'. The article also pointed out that at that time there was no body or corporation with authority to issue qualifications in massage so that the certificates issued by teachers were valueless. Warning was also given about the unsavoury nature of some so called massage establishments which were advertised in the fashionable London papers.

The Society of Trained Masseuses flourished with membership increasing during the First World War. A Royal Charter was granted in 1920 and it became the Chartered Society of Massage and Medical Gymnastics. The name was changed again in 1943 to the Chartered Society of Physiotherapy and state registration followed in 1964. So it was that the use of massage was effectively kept as part of the medical establishment for many years until physiotherapists asserted their professional independence by which time massage was used much less in hospitals.

Following the decline of massage as a treatment for medical conditions there was an increase in its use as part of 'holistic' treatments outside the orthodox medical establishment. Holism is defined in the 1990 Oxford English Dictionary as, 'the treating of the whole person including mental and social factors rather than just symptoms of disease'. Many practitioners are now involved in this alternative view of health care working in clinics, health centres, fitness centres and other places using many different titles.

This recent popularity of complementary therapies has created an interest in massage once again from nurses and other health care professionals. There is a desire by many to return to a more caring role alongside the medical model that has dominated their work in past years.

The skill of massage allows nurses to touch patients therapeutically in a way that allows meaningful communication between them. The importance of touch in caring for people, particularly the elderly and confused, has been shown to promote trust and empathy apart from any physical benefits gained from treatments. Massage is also being used to help patients with conditions believed to be caused by stress and which are made worse by anxiety.

Aromatherapy using massage and aromatic essential oils is also gaining acceptance in some hospitals and clinics where relaxation is seen as a priority. Nurses in training now may be offered some training in massage and in Germany aromatherapy is part of the curriculum for student nurses.

Massage plays a significant part in beauty therapy training and apart from full body massage, is incorporated into many treatments. In facial work, massage movements will be used in cleansing and most other face and skin treatments. In a pedicure treatment, massage movements will be used to apply lotions, to stimulate the circulation and to relax the feet and lower legs. Massage has gradually become a larger part of the beauty therapist's work with the increase in the public's interest in complementary therapies. In 1968 the first full-time nationally recognised course in beauty therapy was offered in a college of further education by the City and Guilds of London Institute and many other organisations now offer full training courses.

Massage and aromatherapy courses will be validated in 1995 by the Health and Beauty Therapy Training Board under the auspices of the National Council for Vocational Qualifications. These competence based courses will allow beauty therapists, nurses and other massage therapists to acquire nationally recognised, free-standing qualifications in both of these skills. It is anticipated that users of this book will be from a variety of backgrounds, and be studying massage and aromatherapy in a variety of contexts. For those readers studying in the beauty therapy or salon setting, a further guide to business practices and procedures can be found in *Health and Beauty Therapy: a Practical Approach for NVQ3* by Jennifer Cartwright and Dawn Mernagh (Stanley Thornes, 1995).

1 The massage therapist in the workplace

After working through this chapter you will be able to:
- ➤ describe a variety of employment opportunities for massage therapists
- ➤ recognise the importance of observing current legislation
- ➤ recognise the importance of personal hygiene.

Body massage is used by massage therapists and beauty therapists for a number of purposes. It can be for relaxation or it may be used in conjunction with creams or lotions that have specific effects on the skin and underlying tissues. Sports therapists use massage to help athletes and sports people to prepare for events and to recover afterwards. Aromatherapists use massage as a method of applying essential oils of plants which have their own specific therapeutic effects. General and localised massage is once again being used in hospitals and hospices as part of therapy for the very ill and the very old, not necessarily for specific medical conditions, but as part of the caring process. Many nurses and professional carers are now training in massage techniques. A great deal of research is taking place designed to see whether recovery rates and the general quality of life can be improved by massage and other complementary therapies.

The types of centre where massage may be carried out and massage therapists employed has increased with the popularity of massage itself.

Beauty salons where facial and body treatments are carried out may include body massage in their slimming or relaxation programmes. Massage, of course, will not of itself make a client lose weight, but does help in making the client more body conscious and may act as an incentive to take more care with diet and exercise.

Salons offering the whole range of treatments are now found not only as small businesses but as part of much larger enterprises. Many large department stores have salons, often with associated treatment spas and facilities for complementary therapies. Hotels, especially those in large towns and holiday resorts, also have salons which offer treatments to an international clientele.

Health farms which were in the past aimed mainly at clients needing to lose weight are now attracting clients in need of relaxation and stress management. Massage is the one therapy that is included in almost every client's regime. Many clients who receive massage for the first time at a health farm become regular clients at beauty salons or other centres. Fitness and sports centres will often have a massage or sports therapist on the premises to work with clients before or after their exercise programme.

Many beauty and massage therapists work on a freelance basis visiting clients in their homes or in hospitals and hospices. Some hospitals now employ massage therapists or specially trained nurses to work principally with patients who have cardiac and psychiatric conditions.

In some offices where there is an effort made to reduce stress at work, the staff may receive a shoulder and neck massage at their desks. Even airlines are now recognising that to offer massage and relaxation treatments in their VIP lounges will attract custom.

Good massage or beauty therapists may well find themselves demonstrating and teaching the lay person to massage as classes are now held in many institutes alongside exercise and yoga classes. In a salon or fitness centre clients may be interested to learn massage techniques to use on their babies and children.

There are many opportunities for a good massage therapist. However, with many more people in training and interest in massage increasing, the work is becoming very competitive. Success as a massage therapist requires dedication and a lot of hard work.

Wherever massage is carried out, the surroundings must be suitable, hygienic and should ensure privacy as far as is possible. Assuming that massage is to be carried out in a beauty salon or similar premises all of the following employment standards apply.

Health and Safety at Work Act 1974

Specifies that the *employer* must:

- safeguard as far as possible the health, safety and welfare of themselves, their employees, contractor's employees and members of the public
- keep all equipment up to standard
- ensure the environment is free from toxic fumes
- have safety equipment checked regularly
- make sure all staff know the safety procedures and provide safety information and training
- ensure safe systems of work.

The *employees* must:

- take reasonable care to avoid injury to themselves and others
- co-operate with others
- not interfere with or misuse anything provided to protect their health and safety.

Fire Precautions Act 1971

- All premises must have fire-fighting equipment in good working order.

* The equipment must be readily available and suitable for the types of fire that are likely to occur.
* Doors should be left unlocked to allow a quick exit in the event of fire.
* Room contents should not obstruct the exits.

Electricity at Work Regulations 1990

Every electrical appliance or piece of equipment must be tested at least once a year by a qualified electrician. A written record must be kept of these tests and be available for inspection by the Health and Safety authority.

COSHH: The Control of Substances Hazardous to Health Act 1989

This act requires employers to identify hazardous substances in the workplace and control people's exposure to them.

The Employer's Liability (Compulsory Insurance) Act 1969

The act requires that employers have everyone on their payroll covered by this insurance and that a current certificate of insurance is displayed at the place of work. The insurance provides cover for claims that might arise when an employee suffers illness or injury as a result of negligence by either the employer or another employee. Employees who are injured as a result of their own negligence are not covered by the act.

Public Liability Insurance

Public liability insurance is not statutary, but is taken out by employers to cover them for claims made by members of the public as a result of injury or damage to personal property caused by the employer or employee at work.

A special Professional Indemnity insurance extends this liability to cover named employees against claims, by clients, of personal injury resulting directly from a treatment.

ACTIVITY	Check your college or salon for safety hazards and note the position and type of any fire-fighting equipment.

When a salon or business is being set up where massage is to be offered commercially, application should be made to the Environmental Services department of the local authority where the establishment is situated. All local authorities issue licences which govern premises and therapists offering certain treatments and some authorities include massage on their list of treatments. Authorities including massage are in the main the metropolitan authorities which have their own bye laws which must be observed. These prescribe standard conditions for special treatment licences, e.g. the Birmingham City Council Act 1990 and the London Local Authorities Act 1991. The licences issued are usually for a year, are charged for and allow for inspection by Environmental Services

Officers who have the authority to fine or cancel the registration of businesses which do not maintain appropriate standards.

Whether a licence is needed or not you must observe basic rules. You must:

* avoid working on clients if you have a contagious disease or infectious illness
* keep your working area clean and tidy
* maintain high standards of hygiene in all aspects of work
* check that the client is suitable for treatment with no contra-indications
* explain the treatment clearly to the client
* take all necessary safety precautions before, during and after treatment
* use correct techniques and never skimp on treatment
* adapt treatment appropriately to suit individual clients
* take care when handling or disposing of substances used in treatments
* remove waste and dispose of it as soon as possible
* keep accurate records of treatments given noting any abnormal reactions or problems.

ACTIVITY

Write to the Environmental Services department of your local authority to find out what conditions must be fulfilled in order to carry out massage treatments in your locality.

GOOD PRACTICE ▷ Massage treatment involves close contact with clients and great care must be taken with personal appearance and hygiene.

* Clothing should be clean and comfortable, allowing adequate room to move while working.
* Jewellery should be kept to an absolute minimum, especially on the hands.
* Hair should be clean, tidy and worn off the face.
* Shoes should have low heels and be comfortable.
* Body and breath odour must be avoided.
* Nails should be clean, short and unvarnished.

REMEMBER

Food and smoke odours cling to clothing and can be very offensive.

KEY TERMS

You need to know what these words mean. Go back through the chapter or check in the glossary to find out.

Therapist	Hygienic	Insurance
Relaxation	Hazards	

2 The working environment

After working through this chapter you will be able to:

> ➤ describe the preferred features of the working area
> ➤ recognise the effect the working environment has on client and therapist
> ➤ describe a variety of beds, couches and supports suitable for use in massage
> ➤ recognise the importance of suitable equipment
> ➤ select appropriate bed, couch or support for the working environment
> ➤ select suitable bed covering and other linen and accessories
> ➤ select massage mediums to suit a variety of clients and massage types.

The working area

As we have seen, a massage therapist may be required to work in many differing environments. However, while massage may be carried out with little or no equipment, a therapist will usually be working in a treatment room specifically set aside for the purpose of massage and related treatments.

Size

A treatment room or cubicle should be large enough to hold the couch and a trolley and to allow the therapist to move freely around the couch.

Decor

A treatment room should be relaxing and welcoming. The working area should preferably have a good supply of natural light. When artificial lighting is needed it should not be too bright and should be indirect so that it does not shine into the client's eyes.

The floor should be of a material that is easily cleaned and maintained, but is not noisy, slippery or too cold.

Temperature and ventilation

The room must be warm enough for the client not to become chilled, but not so warm as to make it uncomfortable for the therapist. It should be ventilated to prevent it becoming stuffy.

In warm climates a quiet method of air-conditioning is ideal, but must not be uncomfortably cooling.

Privacy

The cubicle should be fully enclosed with a material that gives complete privacy to the client. If the cubicle has complete walls rather than curtains, then the door to the cubicle should be able to be completely shut, though it should not be lockable from inside or outside.

Hygiene

Toilet facilities for clients and staff must be readily available. Within the treatment cubicle there should be a washbasin with a supply of soap and disposable towels. There may be showering facilities on the premises depending on the other treatments being carried out, but these are not essential.

Equipment

Trolley

The trolley holds items that will be used during the massage. It should be moveable and have quiet, smooth-running castors. It must be easy to clean. It can be quite small as it is required to hold only the items needed during the treatment.

Table or cupboard

A table or cupboard is required for spare pillows, extra linen and any large items that will not fit onto the trolley.

Massage couch

There is a tremendous variety of suitable couches available for massage therapy, ranging from portable, folding couches suitable for small salons or home visits to the latest 'state of the art' adjustable couches. Whichever couch is used, it must be long and wide enough for clients of varying sizes and must be absolutely secure. There can be nothing worse than lying on a couch that wobbles and squeaks when receiving a massage that should be relaxing!

GOOD PRACTICE ▷ *The height of the couch is important to the therapist; too low and you will have to stoop to work and are quite likely to develop back problems, too high and you have to stretch and will be unable to use your body weight to apply necessary leverage. You should be able to stand by a couch at the correct height and place the flat of your hand on the couch with a straight arm.*

Adjustable couches, although expensive, are the best for a number of reasons; therapists of differing heights can use them, they can be lowered for elderly or disabled clients who might have difficulty in getting onto a normal height couch and they can be used for differing techniques requiring a lower height such as some sports massage manipulations where greater leverage is required.

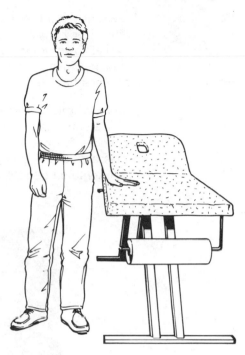

Figure 2.1 *The correct height for a couch*

Couches of all types will have an adjustable backrest and may have other useful features such as a paper roll holder and a breathing hole. They should be covered in an easily cleaned material such as vinyl and be lightly padded for comfort.

Folding/portable couches

Portable couches can be made to order in a variety of heights to suit a particular therapist. They must be stable with legs that can be locked firmly into the open position. They are often supplied with a carrying case to protect the covering during transit. Such couches are portable in

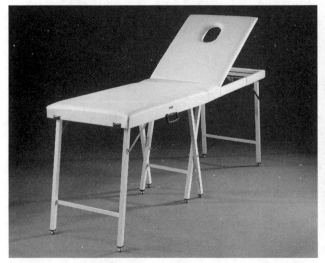

Figure 2.2 *Portable couch – erected*

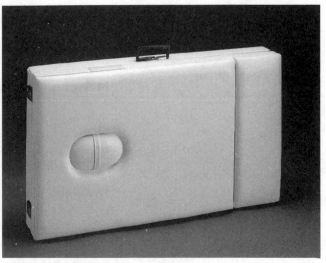

Figure 2.3 *Portable couch – folded*

the sense that they can be folded, but as they weigh 15–17 kg they can be difficult to carry a long way. They are particularly useful for visiting clients in their own homes, for taking to demonstrations or for erecting in a cubicle which is only infrequently used for massage. Some portable couches have legs which can be adjusted to varying heights.

General purpose massage couch

These couches may have a metal or wooden frame and are the basic couches for massage. They may be suitable for treatments other than massage. Some couches are designed to pack flat and can be reassembled quite quickly if needed.

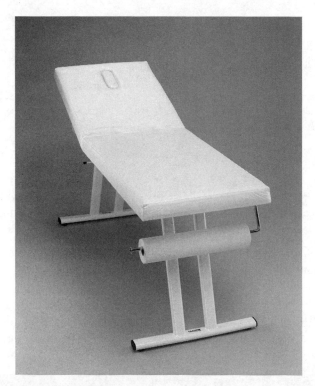

Figure 2.4   *General purpose massage couch*

Multipurpose couch

A multipurpose couch will be suitable for treatments other than massage and will be more versatile than the standard couch. There may be an adjustable foot piece as well as a back support and the central section may allow the shape of the couch to be altered for maximum relaxation and to allow the legs to be raised if necessary.

Hydraulic height-adjustable couch

The couch is raised and lowered by a foot-operated hydraulic pump – similar couches can be operated electrically.

All the couches described above are suitable for a full-body massage and for aromatherapy massage.

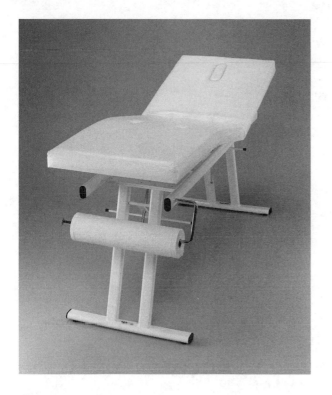

Figure 2.5 *Multi-purpose couch*

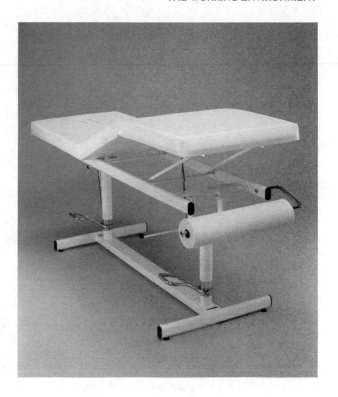

Figure 2.6 *Hydraulic height-adjustable couch*

Sports massage requires an extremely firm surface to be effective and ideally the couch should be adjustable. The most important features of all beds and couches for massage are strength and stability.

For a back massage in the sitting position it may be useful to have a special support which can be propped up on a table to support the client's head and shoulders. This type of support is often used when visiting clients in the office or other workplace.

Steps

A set of steps is useful to allow clients to get on and off the couch more easily. They must be strong and secure and should be stowed away when not in use.

Stool

It is very often convenient to have a stool in the room for the client's or therapist's occasional use during a foot or facial massage.

ACTIVITY	By consulting suppliers and catalogues find out the current cost of each type of couch listed.

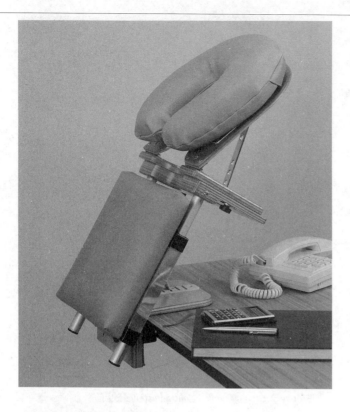

Figure 2.7 *Head and shoulder support*

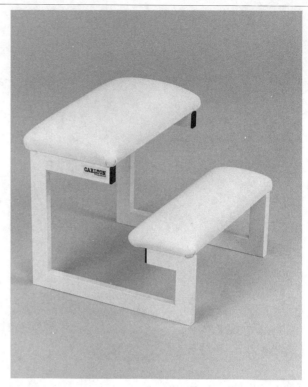

Figure 2.8 *Couch steps*

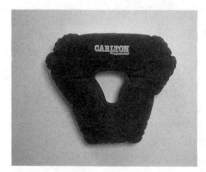

Figure 2.9 *Face cushion*

Accessories

Face cushion

If the couch does not have a breathing hole it will help some clients to use a face cushion which may be inflatable. This allows the client to lie face down in comfort while the therapist is able to work on the back of the neck and shoulders more easily.

Linen

There should be a plentiful supply of fresh, clean linen and this should include:

* covers for the couch made from elasticised towelling or similar material to fit the couch closely
* pillows (small and full size) and pillow covers
* towels of a variety of sizes
* a light blanket.

The couch may be made up with linen in any convenient way. Commonly, it will have the towelling cover in place and two pillows at head level. These will be covered with disposable paper tissue which is usually kept on a roll at the base of the couch.

Two bath size towels can be used to cover the client: one placed across the upper half of the body and the other placed lengthways covering the lower half of the body. This arrangement allows easy access to all parts of the body without too much disturbance.

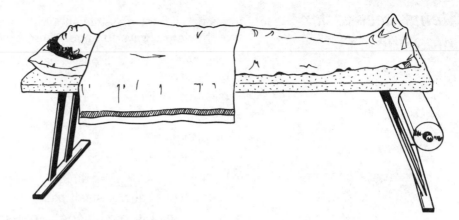

Figure 2.10   *Covering the client*

As the body cools very quickly during massage a blanket should be on hand to cover the client if necessary.

Small pillows or rolled up towels are useful to support parts of the body during the massage, e.g. under the ankle when working on the back of the leg.

Another method of making up the couch is to have a light, flat sheet or blanket on the couch with a covering of disposable paper tissue. The sheet is then folded across the client and folded back to expose each area in turn.

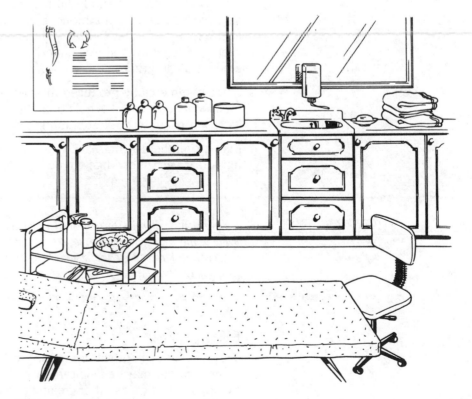

Figure 2.11   *The treatment area*

Items needed for massage

Items needed for massage should be kept on the moveable trolley so that they are always to hand. These should include:

* massage creams and oils in easily cleaned refillable containers which do not spill
* talcum powder
* cologne
* surgical spirit
* facial cleansers
* tissues
* cotton wool balls or small pads
* bowl or small waste bin for used tissue and cotton wool.

Massage creams and oils

There is a vast selection of oils and creams suitable for body massage, ranging from mineral oils, which are cheap and can be bought in bulk, to proprietary brand-name creams and oils, which can be very expensive.

Mineral oils

Mineral oils, such as baby oils, have the disadvantage of not being absorbed easily by the skin. They have the advantage of not going rancid – as vegetable oils may – if kept too long. Mineral oils are particularly suitable for use whilst learning to massage as they are relatively cheap.

Vegetable oils

Any good-quality vegetable oil may be used, such as sunflower, safflower, grapeseed or almond oil. Many therapists use a mixture of oils such as almond oil mixed with a little coconut oil. Care must be taken to keep any vegetable oil fresh and it is a mistake to buy too large an amount at one time.

Some commercially-produced massage oils and creams may be advised for specific purposes such as treating clients with arthritic complaints or localised cellulite or stretch marks.

If an aromatherapy massage is to be carried out, the oils should be mixed for each individual client.

SAFE PRACTICE ▷ *If a client has allergies to perfumed products, a patch test should be carried out before using any perfumed products, i.e. the product should be applied to a small area of skin, for example the inside of the arm, and left for twenty-four hours to see if any reaction occurs.*

Talcum powder

Occasionally a client will prefer not to have oil used on the skin and talcum powder may be an alternative. Talcum does not provide the same level of lubrication as oil or cream but is particularly suitable for deeper, localised manipulations such as those used in sports massage.

Cologne

Cologne is useful to remove excess oil from the skin after the massage should it be necessary and to cleanse the soles of the feet before starting massage.

Surgical spirit

Surgical spirit is used to wipe clean any area of the equipment requiring it. For example, it can be used to clean bowls or to clean away any oil spilt on the trolley.

If facial massage is included in your treatments you will need cleansers to suit the main skin types and products for specialised facial treatments.

When commercial products are used there should be opportunities for the client to discuss and purchase those suitable for home use. They may be displayed in the cubicle as well as in the reception area.

PROGRESS CHECK

List the items which should be placed on the trolley before a massage.

Optional extras

Music

Some therapists like to have music playing while working, however the choice of music is a difficult matter. Many clients will prefer silence and even if they agree to music it is unlikely that their choice will coincide with the therapist's, so a selection of music types should be available. The client could be encouraged to bring their favourite tape. If music is played there should be no attempt to fit the rhythm of the massage to the music.

Refreshment

Clients may be offered some refreshment after the massage and before leaving the salon. Chilled water or fruit juices, coffee or tea, are all suitable.

ACTIVITY

By consulting suppliers, catalogues and local outlets, list as many products as you can which may be used during massage. Compare them in terms of cost, profit margin, packaging and usefulness. Try to assess which products you might select to offer your clients.

┌─ KEY TERMS ───

You need to know what these words mean. Go back through the chapter or check in the glossary to find out.

Environment	Hygiene	Mineral oil
Decor	Portable	Patch test
Temperature		

3 Consultation

After working through this chapter you will be able to:
➤ recognise the importance of client consultation
➤ list the components of a client consultation
➤ recognise the need for tact and understanding when carrying out a consultation
➤ recognise the need for a comprehensive client record system
➤ carry out an effective consultation with regard to massage
➤ describe contra-indications to body massage
➤ describe conditions requiring special care
➤ recognise conditions requiring medical referral.

REMEMBER

*Consultation is a
continuing process.*

Clients may approach a therapist for massage treatments in a number of ways. They may be recommended by another therapist or client or they may contact you as a result of advertising that you have placed. Whatever the case, an initial consultation must be arranged before treatment is carried out. Information is obtained by questioning and by examining the areas to be treated either as part of the initial consultation or later, during treatment.

Aims of a consultation

The aims of a consultation are to:
* find out what the client wants from the treatment
* determine what the client needs from the treatment
* ensure that the client is suitable for treatment
* determine the need for any special care
* establish a good rapport
* answer the client's queries
* agree a treatment plan.

GOOD PRACTICE ▷ *If a treatment or course of treatments is agreed, the client should fully understand the cost and timing of the treatments as no one should be asked to commit themselves to a treatment without fully understanding what is entailed.*

Records of consultations and treatments must be kept. A card or computer system should be devised that allows space for answers to all the questions of the consultation and the results of the examination. A typical record card will contain personal and medical details on one side and a record of attendance and treatments on the other.

When asking personal questions it is important that the therapist maintains a courteous and professional manner and explains the importance of a thorough consultation to the client. The client and therapist should be seated comfortably in an area where they cannot be overheard.

Rather than asking a long list of questions related to the health and lifestyle of the client, questions should be phrased occasionally as open questions to allow the client to answer in their own way and express themselves fully. For example, instead of asking, 'Have you ever had diabetes?' you might ask, 'What sort of health problems have you had?'. Questions that can be answered with a yes or no are closed questions. A question that can't be answered with a yes or no is open. Open questions often begin with how, why, where, what or when.

GOOD PRACTICE ▷ *When carrying out a consultation with elderly or disabled clients, care must be taken to offer help where needed without giving the impression of being patronising or over protective. (A skill that needs a lot of practice!)*

Essential information

Some information such as personal and medical details is essential for the records:

Personal details

* Title.
* Surname.
* Forenames.
* Date of birth or approximate age.
* Address.
* Telephone number at home and at work.

This information is needed in order to contact the client to alter an appointment or to include the client in appropriate future mailshots.

Medical details

* Current medication.
* Current medical treatment.
* Current alternative/complementary treatment.
* Past medical history.

* Past record of surgery and pregnancy.
* General state of health at time of consultation.

The reasons for asking personal and medical questions are to:

* establish the presence or absence of any contra-indications to body massage
* establish whether there are any conditions requiring medical referral
* discover any conditions which require special care to be taken
* discover any localised conditions affecting treatment of that area.

GOOD PRACTICE ▷ *Asking clients questions about their health requires tact and sensitivity. It is usually appropriate to explain to the client why it is necessary to ask the questions. Take care to reassure the client that all records are confidential.*

ACTIVITY

Devise a list of open questions suitable to include in a consultation for a general massage.

Contra-indications

There are few complete contra-indications to a full-body massage, but there are many localised ones. With some contra-indications it may be advisable to consult the client's doctor.

CONTRA-INDICATIONS

to any massage

! When the client is feverish, has an acute infectious disease or is generally unwell.

! When the client is being treated for cancer which may be spread through the lymphatic system, unless the treatment is carried out under medical supervision.

! When the client is under the influence of drink or drugs.

CONTRA-INDICATIONS

to localised massage

! Over a limb where there is a history of thrombosis or phlebitis in the blood vessels.

! Over an area of a skin disorder which may be spread.

! Over an area of inflammation such as a rash or boil.

! Over an area of sunburn.

! Over bruising, cuts, recent scars or abrasions.

! Over recent sprains, fractures or surgical procedures.

REMEMBER

Contra-indication means that the treatment should not be given.

16

! Over a joint that is hot or swollen.

! Over any area of swelling.

! Over very tender or painful muscles.

! Directly over severe varicose veins.

! Directly over moles and warts.

! Over the abdomen during early pregnancy (first three months). Very gentle stroking movements may be used in later stages.

If a client is on any long-term medication then it may be necessary to contact the client's doctor for advice, with the permission of the client.

Conditions where special care should be exercised

* **Diabetes.** In some diabetics circulation is poor, skin sensation may be altered and the skin can become very fragile. The healing process can be very slow, this is especially a problem in the lower leg and foot.

* **Epilepsy.** Most people with epilepsy have their condition well controlled with medication, but special care must be taken not to leave them unattended on a couch.

* **Heart disease or blood pressure disorders.** Very often a client with these conditions will benefit from massage, but the client may need special care. Someone with high blood pressure or heart disease may need to avoid lying flat whereas someone with low blood pressure may feel faint on sitting up and require support.

When a consultation has been completed it is usual for the client to confirm that the information on the card is correct and for them to sign the card to that effect. This is very often a convenient time to agree appointment times and confirm the cost of the treatment. The client should be given the opportunity to ask any questions related to the treatment or the consultation.

<table>
<tr><td>— REMEMBER —

A doctor will not release any information about a patient unless the patient has given the doctor permission in writing.</td></tr>
</table>

ACTIVITY	Design a record card suitable for use by a massage therapist.

Client records must be kept safely in a secure place and updated whenever the client attends for treatment. A full record of treatments given, products used and any special requirements needed should be kept and referred to. If records are kept on computer then the Data Protection Act applies and the therapist should conform to the requirements of the act.

Data Protection Act

The Data Protection Act gives clients the right to see personal data held on computer about them and to get it corrected if it is wrong. Computer users who keep information about individuals must, by law, appear in the Data Protection Register.

ACTIVITY

Working with a partner, role-play a consultation with a new client. Imagine that the client has never had massage before but has been recommended to you by another client. Ask a colleague to watch the role-play and give feedback on how successful you were in putting the client at ease and eliciting the correct information.

KEY TERMS

You need to know what these words mean. Go back through the chapter or check in the glossary to find out.

Rapport
Open questions
Closed questions

Personal details
Medical details

Medication
Contra-indications

4 Massage and the systems of the body

After working through this chapter you will be able to:
- ➤ describe the main features of the body systems relevant to body massage
- ➤ describe the main functions of these systems
- ➤ describe the main effects of massage on these body systems
- ➤ relate any contra-indications of massage to these systems and their structure and function
- ➤ describe the effects of stress on the body
- ➤ relate the effects of massage to the management of stress
- ➤ relate any specific effects of aromatherapy massage on these systems.

The systems of the body relevant to body massage

a) Integumentary system (skin and its derivatives, such as nails and hair).
b) Musculo-skeletal system (bones, joint and muscles).
c) Circulatory system.
d) Lymphatic system.
e) Nervous system.
f) Respiratory system.
g) Digestive system.
h) Renal system.
i) Endocrine system.
j) Immune system.

Integumentary system

The integumentary system is the name given to the skin and its derivatives (hair, nails and glands). The skin is the part of the integumentary system which forms the outer surface of the body and is the part of the body which is immediately affected by massage. The skin envelopes the body and is the largest organ in the body, covering on an adult an area of approximately two square metres. Skin varies in thickness in different parts of the body from very thin skin, about 0.05 mm thick, on the eyelids and lips to much thicker skin on the soles of the feet or palms of the hands, which is approximately 3.5 mm at its thickest.

Structure
The skin is composed of two main layers – the epidermis and the deeper dermis.
The epidermis itself consists of five layers, each called a stratum.

19

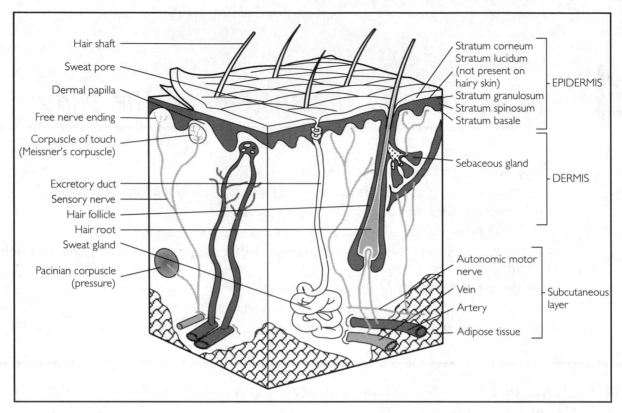

Figure 4.1 *Sectional view of the skin*

Stratum corneum
This is the superficial layer. It is made of many rows of flattened, dead cells which contain the tough protein keratin. The outer cells of this layer are shed regularly and some of them will be rubbed off by massage, especially if a body-peeling cream is used to prepare the skin for massage.

Stratum lucidum
This is a clear layer formed by three or four rows of clear, flat, dead cells and is found only in the palms of the hands and soles of the feet where it acts to resist friction.

Stratum granulosum
This is a layer of two to three rows of cells that contain a substance involved in the formation of keratin.

Stratum spinosum
This is a layer of eight to ten rows of many-sided cells fitting closely together. The stratum spinosum, together with the deepest layer of the epidermis helps to form new cells.

Stratum basale
This deepest layer of the epidermis is a single row of oblong, columnar cells that divide continually. As the cells of the stratum basale multiply, they push up to the surface, progressively becoming part of the upper

layers of the epidermis until they die and are shed from the stratum corneum. In this way the epidermis is replaced regularly every few weeks.

The dermis is the deeper layer of the skin and is much thicker than the epidermis. It contains the connective tissue which gives the skin its elasticity and strength as well as hair follicles, blood vessels, nerves and glands.

The upper part of the dermis has finger-like projections that extend into the epidermis. This papillary layer of the dermis contains nerve endings which are sensitive to touch, some called Meissner's corpuscles sense light touch while others called Pacinian corpuscles are sensitive to deep pressure so that it is here that the difference between various massage movements are registered.

The dermis also contains blood and lymph vessels, nerves, hair follicles, sweat glands and collagenous and elastic connective tissue fibres.

The elastic connective tissues in the skin become less efficient during the ageing process. It is this loss of elasticity which explains why the skin of older people is looser and more wrinkled. This laxity of the skin is one of the factors that must be taken into consideration when massaging an older client, as too deep or brisk movements could be very uncomfortable.

ACTIVITY	Pinch the skin on the back of your hand, release it and note how long it takes to return to normal. Ask a number of people of different ages to do the same and note the differences in elasticity.

Hair grows from a root deep in the dermis. The shaft of the hair passes through the epidermis to project above the surface of the skin. It is present on most of the body areas covered by massage except the soles of the feet and palms of the hands. Hair varies in length and texture on different parts of the body. In its normal position, hair lies at an angle to the skin and where possible massage strokes should be in the direction of this natural lie of the hair, especially if the hair is long or very vigorous.

The dermis contains the blood vessels that supply the skin. These capillaries dilate or constrict in response to external factors – mainly heat and cold. When the capillaries are dilated more blood flows close to the surface of the skin and when they are constricted less blood flows. Depending on the amount of pigment in the skin, the dilation and constriction of capillaries in the dermis may affect the skin colour temporarily. Warm skin looks redder than cool skin. This will be noted in massage treatments as the massage warms the skin. The reddening is called erythema.

Lymph capillaries are blind-ended tubes that begin in spaces between cells and are present in the deeper part of the skin. More mention will be made of these in the section on the lymphatic system (p. 37).

There are two types of gland present in the dermis which have openings to the surface of the skin. These are the sweat glands and the sebaceous glands.

Sweat glands are found over the surface of the body and are most numerous on the soles of the feet and the palms of the hands. They are also very numerous on the forehead and armpits. Each gland has a coiled part in the dermis and a tube leading to a pore on the surface. They produce a thin, watery, salty fluid, commonly known as perspiration or sweat. Their main function is to regulate body temperature by producing sweat in response to heat. The body cools as the sweat evaporates. A client who becomes very warm during a massage may sweat excessively and this may result in the therapist's hands slipping too much. It is also possible that the therapist's hands may sweat too much with the same result. Excessive sweating on the palms of the hands can occur if the therapist is nervous for any reason and is often a problem for a student. With time and confidence the problem diminishes.

The second type of gland is the sebaceous gland. These glands are situated in the hair follicles and produce an oily liquid called sebum. Sebaceous glands are not found on the soles of the feet or palms of the hand and are quite small in the skin covering most of the trunk and limbs. They are large in the skin of the upper chest, face and neck. The sebum produced by the glands keeps the skin and hair soft and supple. The production of sebum is often stimulated by massage. Beneath the dermis is a layer of connective tissue containing adipose tissue.

Adipose tissue

This is a type of loose connective tissue containing cells which are specially adapted to store fat. Adipose tissue is found under the skin and around organs. It acts as a reserve of food and as it is a poor conductor of heat, helps to maintain body temperature by preventing heat loss.

Massage is often said to affect adipose tissue by softening hard fat under the skin and helping it to disperse into the deeper tissue and circulatory system. Many massage creams are also said to help with the dispersal of subcutaneous fat.

The distribution of the fat layer under the skin varies according to sex, age and lifestyle. Women tend to have a thicker layer of adipose tissue than men, giving the female body a softer outline with the muscles being less obvious. After the menopause women tend to put on weight in the more masculine pattern, i.e. on the waist and abdomen rather than the hips and thighs

Absorption

For many years biologists thought that the skin formed an impervious barrier to external substances, but more recent research shows that most chemicals placed on the skin can be absorbed to some degree. Some chemicals are absorbed only into the skin and some penetrate across the skin to enter the bloodstream and travel around the body. In some cases this effect can be beneficial. For example, drugs for the treatment of heart and endocrine disorders can be delivered by means of patches containing the drugs being placed on the skin. In other cases the absorption of chemicals through the skin may be very harmful, which is why industrial workers handling hazardous materials such as mercury will wear protective clothing.

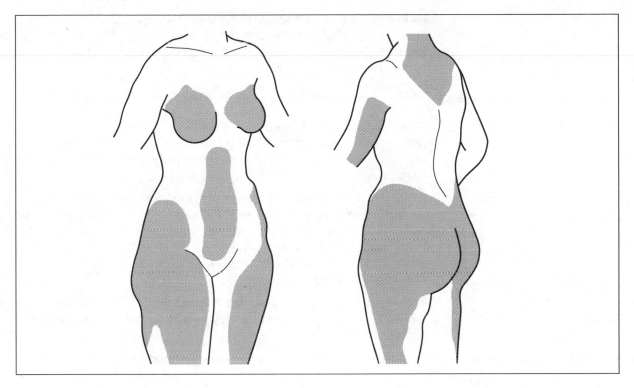

Figure 4.2 *Fat distribution (female)*

There are many factors which determine how much of a chemical penetrates the skin. Some of these factors are:

* the amount and concentration of the chemical applied
* the length of time the chemical is in contact with the skin
* the skin's temperature and moisture content
* the concentration of hair follicles and sweat ducts in the skin in the area where the chemical is applied
* whether the skin is damaged in any way.

All of these are likely to affect the absorption of substances such as aromatherapy oils.

Although there is little information on the absorption of essential oils as such, there has been research on the skin penetration of fragrance chemicals. This research shows that absorption is greater over areas of thinner, more delicate skin, such as that on the face and eyelids, and less on the thicker skin on the palms of the hands and soles of the feet. Children's skin is more permeable than adults'.

The two major factors governing the level of absorption of such chemicals by the skin appear to be the strength of the dose applied and the size of the area to which it is applied. Massage and heat may also encourage absorption as will covering the area with clothes or towels.

Allergy

Substances applied to the skin may cause the skin to react allergically against the substance. The reaction of some of the cells of the dermis is to release histamine, causing the tissue to become red, warm and swollen. The first contact with the substance may leave the tissue sensitised so that later contact can cause a more severe and generalised reaction. Once a person has become sensitised to a substance it must be completely avoided.

SAFE PRACTICE ▷ *Clients should always be asked if they are allergic to any substances used in products being applied to the skin. If there is any doubt, perform a patch test. Apply some of the substance to a small patch of skin and check for any reaction after 24 hours.*

Aromatherapy products which contain the essential oils of plants are often considered safe because they are pure and natural. However they are potent, concentrated, natural chemicals and some can be toxic. For example, the oil from the pennyroyal plant contains a liver toxin and cinnamon bark oil can cause allergic skin reactions. The contra-indications of individual oils must be checked before use on the skin.

The commonest way of applying these essential oils is by massage which increases the flow of blood to the area and this may enhance absorption of the substances into the body.

Photosensitivity
Certain chemicals cause the skin to react more strongly than usual when exposed to sunlight. The best known of these used in perfumery and aromatherapy is oil of bergamot. The result can be 'sunburn' or a rash after a very short exposure to ultra-violet light. It follows that any product containing a photosensitiser should not be applied to the skin before exposure to natural or artificial sunlight (e.g. a sunbed).

Effects of massage on skin

- Desquamation – the removal of dead cells from the surface of the skin – improving skin texture.
- Stimulation of sweat and sebaceous glands giving a 'cleansing' effect.
- Improving the circulation to the skin, increasing nourishment and assisting the removal of waste products.
- Warming the skin, temporarily producing an erythema.

Products used on the skin during massage will have their own specific effects.

CONTRA-INDICATIONS to massage over a particular area of skin.

! Any skin infection.

! Severe bruising.

! Breaks in the skin.

! Moles and warts.

! Sunburn.

! Any contra-indication to specific products used.

Musculo-skeletal system

The skeleton is constructed from dense connective tissue, as are the ligaments which attach bone to bone at the joints and the tendons which attach muscles to bone. Massage over tendons and ligaments can help to keep them flexible and is of particular value in a sports massage.

Massage is unlikely to have a direct effect on the bony skeleton or the joints, but may have an indirect effect through stimulating the blood supply. It is important for therapists to know the position of the parts of the skeleton and to recognise those superficial areas of the skeleton which protrude in some clients and which require special care during massage. During a sports massage, knowledge of the whole musculo-skeletal system is of great importance. In a sports massage the massage is often aimed at specific problem areas with the massage strokes following the direction of the muscle fibres or being directed across them depending on the effects required.

The skeleton

The skeleton forms the framework of the body and is formed of bone and cartilage. Bones are attached to each other at joints where they are held together by ligaments and muscles.

Functions of the skeleton

The skeleton:

* supports the soft tissues of the body
* protects structures such as the brain, spinal cord and heart
* stores salts, such as calcium
* produces blood cells in the marrow of the bones.

Structure of the skeleton

The skeleton is made up of 206 bones. It is divided into two main parts, the axial skeleton and the appendicular skeleton.

The axial skeleton is made up of bones which lie around the centre of the body. The bones of the axial skeleton are listed in Table 4.1 below.

The appendicular skeleton consists of the bones of the upper and lower limbs and the bones that attach them to the axial skeleton, the pectoral and pelvic girdles. The bones of the appendicular skeleton are listed in Table 4.2 below.

In massage, the outline of the skeleton is followed and bony points that are not covered by soft tissue must be treated lightly. Some points can be very painful if deep movements are applied. As the hands are very sensitive, the difference between soft tissue such as fat or muscle and hard, bony tissue should be easily felt and massage to the obvious bony points should be avoided.

	Bones	Number of bones
Head	Cranium	8
	Face	14
	Ear	6
	Hyoid (in the throat)	1
Thorax	Sternum	1
	Ribs	24
Spine	Vertebrae	26

Table 4.1 *Bones of the axial skeleton*

Components		Number of bones
Pectoral girdle	Clavicle	2
	Scapula	2
Upper limbs		60
Pelvic girdle	Pelvic bones	2
Lower limbs		60

Table 4.2 *Bones of the appendicular skeleton*

CONTRA-INDICATIONS

to massage and points of special care related to the skeleton.

❗ Massage should not be applied over a fractured bone until it is completely healed.

❗ If metal plates or pins have been inserted in the bones, care must be taken over the area and medical advice sought.

❗ Any condition under medical care.

❗ Any unexplained bone pain.

ACTIVITY

Find the following prominent bony points on Figures 4.3 and 4.4 and on yourself from the head down.

● Base of the occipital bone.

● Mastoid process.

● 7th cervical vertebra.

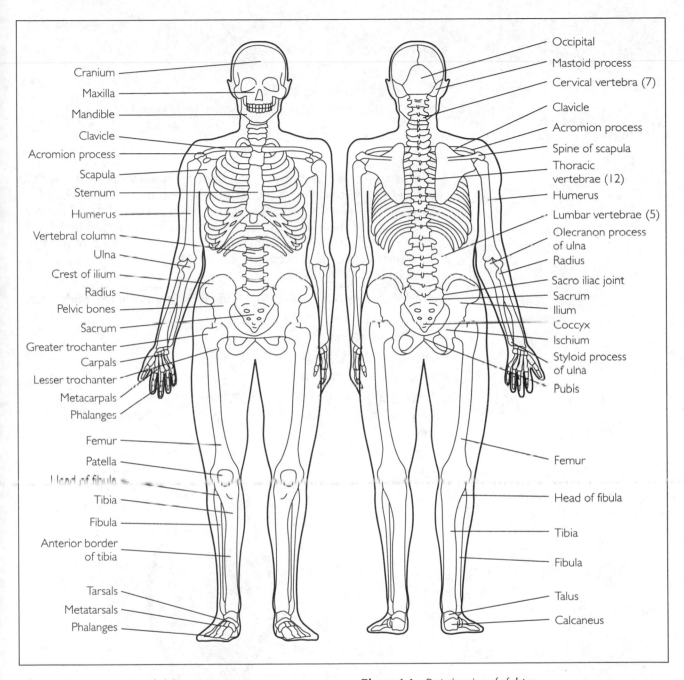

Cranium
Maxilla
Mandible
Clavicle
Acromion process
Scapula
Sternum
Humerus
Vertebral column
Ulna
Crest of ilium
Radius
Pelvic bones
Sacrum
Greater trochanter
Carpals
Lesser trochanter
Metacarpals
Phalanges
Femur
Patella
Head of fibula
Tibia
Fibula
Anterior border of tibia
Tarsals
Metatarsals
Phalanges

Occipital
Mastoid process
Cervical vertebra (7)
Clavicle
Acromion process
Spine of scapula
Thoracic vertebrae (12)
Humerus
Lumbar vertebrae (5)
Olecranon process of ulna
Radius
Sacro iliac joint
Sacrum
Ilium
Coccyx
Ischium
Styloid process of ulna
Pubis
Femur
Head of fibula
Tibia
Fibula
Talus
Calcaneus

Figure 4.3 *Anterior view of skeleton*

Figure 4.4 *Posterior view of skeleton*

- Clavicle.
- Spine of the scapula.
- Acromion process.
- Olecranon process (take care here, a nerve crosses the elbow – commonly called the funny bone).
- Styloid process of the ulna.
- Crest of the ilium.

27

- Sacro-iliac joint.
- Greater trochanter of the femur.
- Patella.
- Anterior border of the tibia.
- Head of the fibula (take care, another nerve crosses here).

Joints

A joint is a place where bones in the body meet. At some joints, such as those of the adult skull, the bones inter-lock so that there is no movement between them. At other joints, such as those formed between the vertebrae of the spine, the bones are loosely connected by flexible cartilage which allows only limited movement. A third kind of joint allows free movement between the bones. This kind of joint is known as a synovial joint.

Synovial joints are the most numerous type of joint in the body. They have a number of common features.

- Muscles surround the joint.
- Ligaments hold the bones together
- A capsule of connective tissue encloses the joint.
- A synovial membrane lines the capsule.
- Synovial fluid is produced by the synovial membrane to lubricate the joint.
- Cartilage covers the bony surfaces where they meet.

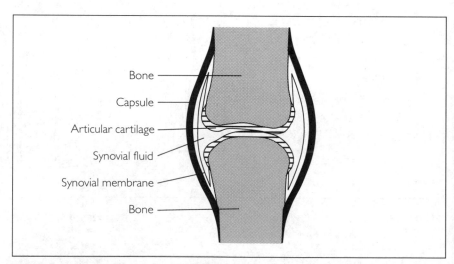

Figure 4.5 *Section through a synovial joint*

Massage affects the joints indirectly by stimulating the circulation and lymphatic flow in the region of the joint. Some therapists may include a series of passive movements in a massage treatment. A passive movement is one where the therapist moves a joint through a range of movements while the client is relaxed. They are thought to improve and maintain the mobility of the joints and aid the circulation.

CONTRA-INDICATIONS to massage related to the joints.

! Over any swelling of a joint when the cause is not known.

! Over any joint that is hot or painful.

! Over any joint where a strain or sprain is suspected.

ACTIVITY Find out as much as possible about various forms of arthritis, e.g. rheumatoid arthritis, osteo-arthritis and ankylosing spondylitis.

Muscle tissue

There are three types of muscle tissue; skeletal, cardiac and visceral. Skeletal muscle tissue forms the muscles that are felt during massage.

Muscle tissue makes up 40 to 50% of body weight.

* It is excitable in that it receives and responds to stimuli in the form of nerve impulses.
* It can contract, shortening and thickening when stimulated.
* It can be stretched.
* It is elastic, returning to its original shape after contracting or being stretched.

Skeletal (voluntary) muscle is attached to bones by means of connective tissue such as tendons and, as its name suggests, it is under voluntary control. For a muscle fibre to contract it must first be stimulated by a nerve cell.

Individual muscles or groups of muscle fibres have their own nerve and blood supplies. Muscle contraction requires a good blood supply to bring oxygen and nutrients to provide energy and to remove the waste products of contraction. By contracting, skeletal muscles perform three important functions. They:

* move parts of the body
* maintain the upright posture of the body
* produce heat – a by-product of the work done by the muscle in contracting.

Some massage movements, particularly tapotement movements such as hacking, can cause muscle fibres to contract. This repetitive contraction and relaxation of the muscle fibres stimulates blood flow in the same way that exercise does. Hacking has been shown to be much more effective than any other massage stroke in increasing blood flow to muscles.

Muscles tend to work in groups and when one group of muscles works to produce a movement there will be an opposing group of muscles which has to relax to allow the movement to happen. For example the muscles in the front of the upper arm (the biceps) contract to bend the elbow, but the elbow would not be able to move unless the muscles on the back of the arm (the triceps) relax.

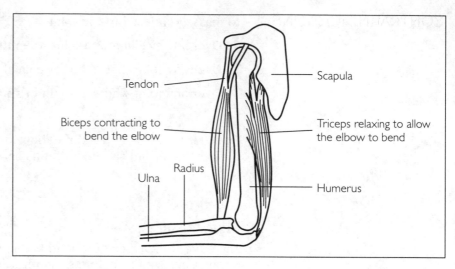

Figure 4.6 *Muscles of the upper arm*

ACTIVITY

Bend your arm at the elbow against some resistance, e.g. with your hand under the edge of a table. With the other hand feel the biceps and the triceps muscles and note the difference.

Muscle tone

At any given time some fibres in a muscle are contracted while others are relaxed. Not enough fibres are contracted to produce movement, but this helps to maintain posture without any noticeable effort. This partial muscle contraction is called muscle tone and the term is commonly used to describe the firmness or flabbiness of muscle. Good muscle tone is achieved and maintained by exercise, but some massage movements, such as hacking, that stretch muscle fibres may help to maintain the tone of superficial muscles. Massage is adapted to suit clients with different levels of muscle tone so that the massage used on an elderly client who exercises infrequently will be very different from that used on a sportsman or sportswoman who has firm, well-toned muscles. It is important that a therapist develops hands which are sensitive to these differences.

Muscle fatigue

During gentle or moderate exercise, muscles are able to obtain sufficient energy aerobically by oxidising glucose in the body. As exercise increases, there is not enough oxygen available and energy is produced from glucose anaerobically. A waste product called lactic acid is produced when muscles produce energy anaerobically. Lactic acid builds up in the muscles, slowing them down and sometimes causing cramp. One of the purposes of massage after exercise is to aid the removal of lactic acid from the muscles.

Massage is often used to relax muscles, either by general massage to bring about relaxation of the whole body or by working on specific muscles, such as those used in particular movements. In either case a knowledge of the shape and position of the superficial muscles of the

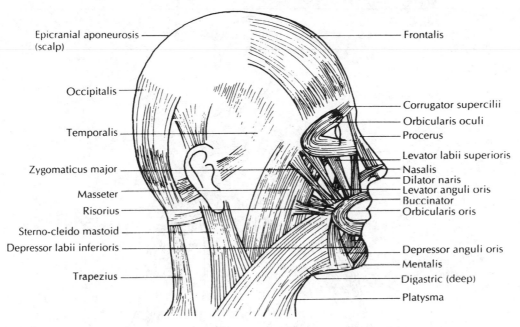

Figure 4.7 *Facial muscles*

body is important. In sports massage in particular the massage strokes will be directed along the length of muscle fibres or across them depending on the effects required.

Some muscles are small and delicate, such as the muscles of the face, and here in particular massage movements should follow the direction of the muscle fibres where possible.

Effects of massage on muscle tissue

* stimulate the blood supply which brings fresh nutrients and oxygen to the muscles and removes waste products
* help to reduce muscle fatigue
* help to maintain the elasticity of muscle fibres
* help to reduce adhesions in muscle tissue which may have developed following injury.

CONTRA-INDICATIONS to massage related to the muscles.

! Over muscles which are painful.

! Over muscles which are tender.

--- KEY TERMS ---

You need to know what these words mean. Go back through the section or check in the glossary to find out.

Appendicular	Ligaments	Synovial
Axial	Muscle tone	Tendons
Cartilage		

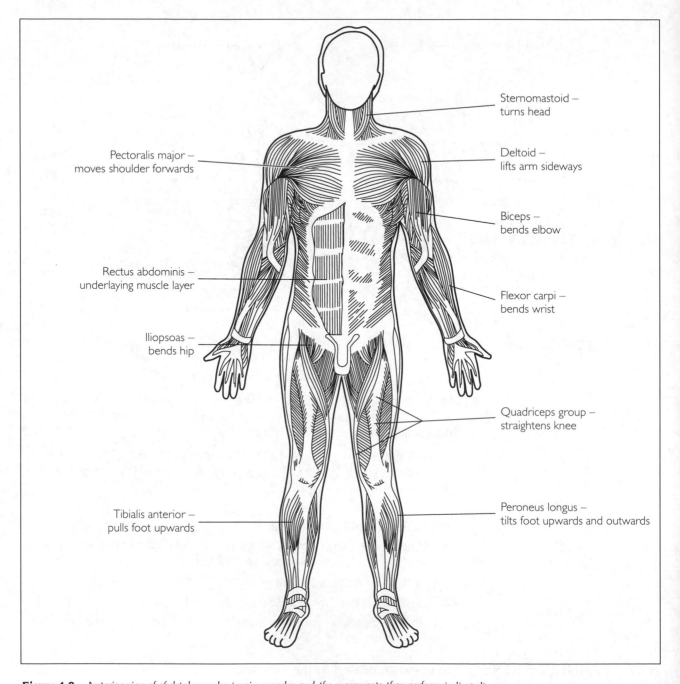

Figure 4.8 *Anterior view of skeletal muscles (main muscles and the movements they perform indicated)*

Circulatory system

Blood is a complex fluid consisting of red and white blood cells, platelets and the liquid plasma. The functions of blood are to:

* transport oxygen from the lungs to the cells of the body
* transport carbon dioxide from the cells of the body to the lungs
* transport nutrients from the digestive organs to the cells
* transport waste products from the cells to the kidneys, lungs and sweat glands

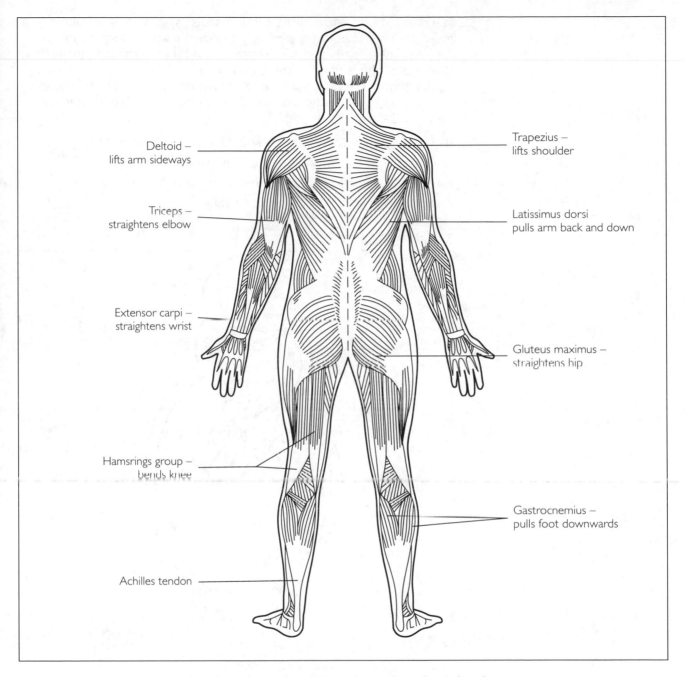

Figure 4.9 *Posterior view of skeletal muscles (main muscles and the movements they perform indicated)*

- transport hormones from the endocrine glands to the cells
- transport enzymes to various cells
- regulate the pH of the body
- help to regulate body temperature
- regulate the water content of cells
- protect the body against infection and toxic substances.

33

The heart is the centre of the cardiovascular system. It is a hollow, muscular organ about the size of a clenched fist. It is located in the centre of the chest between the lungs and is tilted to the left. Its function is to pump blood through the blood vessels of the body. It acts as a double pump; the right side pumps deoxygenated blood to the lungs to receive oxygen while the left side pumps oxygenated blood from the lungs to the rest of the body.

Blood is carried around the body in blood vessels. These are:

* arteries – which carry blood from the heart
* veins – which carry blood to the heart
* capillaries – which link arteries to veins

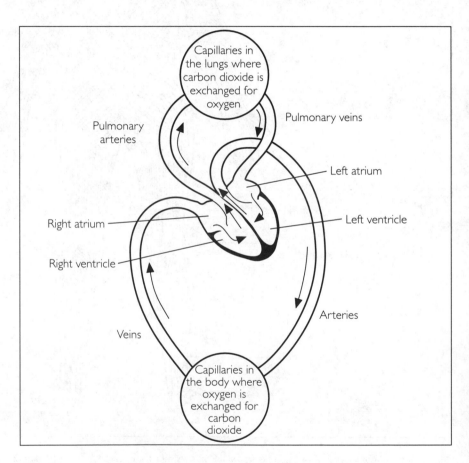

Figure 4.10 *The double circulatory system of the body*

The heart pumps oxygenated blood into large arteries which then branch into smaller and smaller arteries. The smallest of these arteries are called arterioles and they reach to all parts of the body. The arterioles link with the tiny capillaries in the tissues which in turn connect with the smallest veins, called venules. Venules join together to form veins which return the blood to the heart.

Arteries and veins differ in structure. Arteries have thicker walls which contain muscle fibres to help control the flow of blood through them. Every time the heart beats, it pushes blood through the arteries and it can be felt in large arteries as the pulse, e.g. the radial pulse at the wrist.

Veins have thinner walls than arteries and have valves to prevent the blood flowing backwards. Blood is kept moving in veins by the squeezing action of surrounding muscles contracting and relaxing and to a lesser degree by the pressure in the arteries pushing blood through the capillaries and veins.

Varicose veins is a condition where the valves fail to keep the blood in the veins from flowing backwards and the walls of the veins bulge, becoming very prominent. They are often caused by standing for long periods without sufficient muscular activity and also occur in some women during pregnancy. The skin over the region of severe varicose veins is often thin and papery and if damaged may break down to form ulcers. Care must always be taken when working over such an area.

Occasionally clots may form in the blood in places that cause problems. Examples of this are the clots which can form in the arteries of the heart muscle (coronary arteries) which can cause heart attacks, and the clots which can form in the arteries to the brain which can cause strokes.

Clots may also form in veins, particularly in the legs in both superficial and deep veins. When clots are formed in superficial veins, the condition is called thrombo phlebitis and is often associated with varicose veins. The area is usually warm, swollen and is very tender and painful. When a clot, or thrombus, forms in a deep vein the condition is called deep venous thrombosis. This condition may follow surgery, hormonal treatment or travel in cramped conditions, such as a long air flight where movement of the legs is limited. There will be localised swelling in the limb affected but there is often no pain unless the area is probed quite deeply.

SAFE PRACTICE ▷ *Neither thrombo phlebitis nor deep venous thrombosis should ever be treated by massage. Localised swelling, especially in the calf of one leg, should always be referred to a doctor. If massage is carried out there is a risk that the clot may be moved or broken up. The clot, or fragments of it, may then travel through the circulatory system to the lungs where they may cause great harm. If the client has had either of these conditions in the past, then clearance should be sought from the client's doctor before treating the area.*

Massage strokes such as effleurage can help the return of blood through the veins as the strokes are performed in the direction of venous flow towards the heart.

ACTIVITY

Firmly stroke the inside of your arm upwards from wrist to elbow. Note the emptying of the superficial veins followed by rapid filling.

Blood pressure

The pressure of the blood in the arteries and arterioles reaches a peak when the heart contracts; this is called the systolic blood pressure. It gradually decreases to the minimum allowed by the elasticity of the artery walls, the diastolic blood pressure, just before the next contraction. Blood pressure is always recorded as two figures, the systolic pressure being shown over the diastolic pressure, e.g. 120/80. The figures represent the pressures measured in millimetres of mercury.

Blood pressure varies with age, sex and weight. It tends to increase with age. It may be raised for short periods by exercise or stress and anxiety and be lowered by rest and contentment.

High blood pressure

When people have a blood pressure that is at a continuously high level they will be at a greater risk of strokes, heart attacks and kidney damage. Consequently many clients with high blood pressure will be taking medication to modify it. Clients with high blood pressure may be more comfortable if they do not lie completely flat during treatment.

Low blood pressure

Blood pressure must be sufficient to pump blood to the brain when the body is in the upright position. If it is not, then the person will faint. Some people with low blood pressure may feel faint when sitting up suddenly from the lying position.

Effects of massage on the circulatory system

* Speeds the flow of blood through the veins.
* Causes dilation of superficial capillaries producing skin erythema.
* Stimulates the supply of fresh, oxygenated blood to the superficial tissues.
* Stimulates the removal of waste products from the superficial tissues.
* Reduces the viscosity, or stickiness, of the blood.
* May reduce blood pressure.

CONTRA-INDICATIONS

to massage related to the circulatory system.

! Over an area which has, or has had in the past, a deep venous thrombosis or thrombo phlebitis.

! Over obvious varicose veins.

! Over an area of swelling or tenderness.

ACTIVITY

Find out what the 'normal' range of blood pressure is.

KEY TERMS

You need to know what these words mean. Go back through the section or check in the glossary to find out.

Arterioles	Hormones	Thrombus
Capillaries	pH value	Venule
Enzymes	Toxic	

The lymphatic system

The lymphatic system supplements the circulatory system by removing excess fluid from the tissues. It consists of:

- lymph nodes, often called lymph glands, which are linked together by
- lymph vessels and capillaries, large and small thin walled tubes scattered through the tissues of the body
- lymphatic tissue, found in associated organs such as the tonsils, adenoids, spleen and liver.

The lymphatic capillaries collect excess fluid from the body along with any bacteria, viruses and other particles that need removing from the tissues. This fluid is called lymph and passes through the capillaries which join to form larger lymphatic vessels. The lymph passes through lymph nodes where the unwanted particles are filtered out and removed. Eventually the vessels join to become two large vessels which empty their contents back into the main circulatory system at the veins in the base of the neck.

The functions of the lymphatic system are to:

- remove excess fluid from the tissues
- filter out unwanted material
- help to absorb fat from around the intestine
- produce lymphocytes (a type of white blood cell) which destroy bacteria and viruses
- produce antibodies as part of the body's immune system.

Lymph glands, or nodes, sometimes swell when there is an infection in the locality because the nodes make large quantities of lymphocytes with which to fight the infection. Thus the nodes of the neck can swell when there is a throat infection. Infection can also travel along lymphatic vessels until a group of nodes is reached. For example, if a hand is infected the nodes in the elbow or armpit may swell. Other matter, such as cancer cells, may be spread along the lymphatic pathways, therefore surgery or radiotherapy for localised cancer may be targeted at particular lymph nodes.

More commonly, sluggish lymphatic drainage in part of the system will lead to puffiness, often called water retention. The feet and ankles may be swollen in the evening and some people will become uncomfortable in tight clothes as the day passes.

Effects of massage on the lymphatic system

- Stimulates the flow of lymph in the lymphatic capillaries and superficial vessels.
- Reduces generalised swelling in the tissues.
- Stimulates the absorption of waste matter.

CONTRA-INDICATIONS to massage related to the lymphatic system.

! Over swollen lymph nodes.

■ Over an infected vessel (seen as a red line under the skin leading to swollen nodes).

■ Cancer – unless recommended by a doctor.

Massage is often carried out specifically to stimulate superficial lymphatic drainage of part of, or the whole of, the body. When this is the case, strokes will be in the direction of lymphatic drainage towards the nearest lymph nodes.

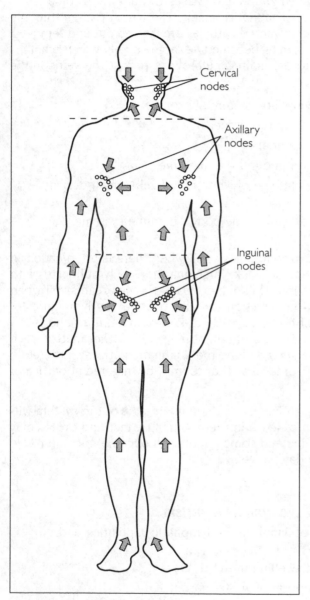

Figure 4.11 *Anterior view of superficial drainage in the lymphatic system*

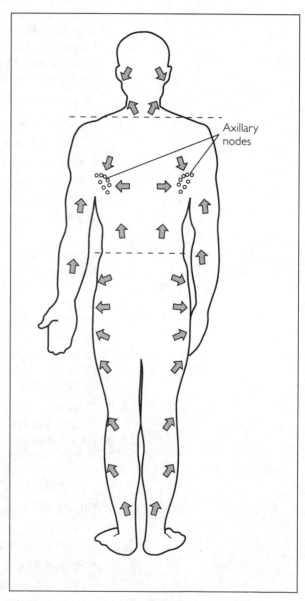

Figure 4.12 *Posterior view of superficial drainage in the lymphatic system*

KEY TERMS

You need to know what these words mean. Go back through the section or check in the glossary to find out.

Lymph   Lymphocytes   Lymph nodes

Nervous system

The function of the nervous system is to carry messages around the body, controlling and co-ordinating other systems. It stimulates movement and together with the endocrine system maintains home-ostasis. It senses change inside and outside the body, interprets those changes and initiates actions to deal with them.

The nervous system consists of:

* the central nervous system which is the control centre – the brain and spinal cord
* the peripheral nervous system – the nerves which carry messages to and from the central nervous system.

All sensations from the body will be relayed by the peripheral nervous system to the central nervous system to be interpreted and acted upon.

The nerves which carry messages from the central nervous system may go to the skeletal muscles to produce movement which is under voluntary control or to involuntary muscle, cardiac muscle and to glands. This latter part is called the autonomic nervous system and operates without conscious control.

Sensations

A stimulus of some kind will be sensed by a sense organ or receptor and converted into nerve impulses which are conveyed to the sensory part of the brain. The stimulus may be light, heat, smell, or touch and pressure as in the case of massage.

The receptors or sense organs are parts of the body that contain cells that are sensitive to stimuli, for example cells in the eyes, ears , nose and skin.

Receptors called exteroceptors are sensitive to stimuli originating outside the body and transmit sensations of hearing, sight, smell, touch, pressure, temperature and pain. These exteroceptors are located near the surface of the body. Receptors called interoceptors are sensitive to stimuli originating inside the body such as pain, pressure, taste, fatigue, hunger and thirst. Interoceptors are situated deeper in the body. Receptors called proprioceptors are situated in muscles, tendons and joints and in the inner ear and are sensitive to the position of parts of the body.

When a stimulus is applied continuously its effect becomes less with time. This is especially true of touch sensations, for example, when you put on your clothes you are aware of them, but the sensation gradually fades. This is called sensory adaptation and has an important role in

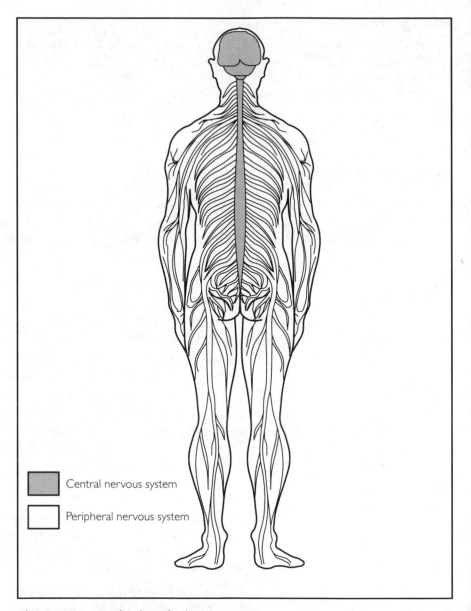

Figure 4.13 *Central and peripheral nervous systems*

massage as the client will gradually become accustomed to the feeling of being massaged and be able to relax as this adaptation takes place.

The most obvious sensations relating to massage are those received by receptors in the skin and the connective tissue just under the skin. These receptors are found all over the body, but are denser in some parts than others. Areas with many receptors will be much more sensitive than areas with fewer receptors. Skin receptors for fine touch are found in the top of the dermis and include Meissner's corpuscles which are most numerous in the fingertips, palms of the hands and soles of the feet. Receptors for deep pressure are deep in the dermis and are called Pacinian corpuscles. They are less sensitive to variations than the fine touch receptors.

The receptors in the skin are important to the therapist and the client. Too light a touch can be very irritating to a client who needs a deep massage and similarly too deep pressure can be painful. The therapist should use the very sensitive palms of the hands to register the reaction of the client which would probably be to tense the muscles in response to discomfort. The massage can then be adapted accordingly.

The autonomic nervous system carries messages from the central nervous system to control and regulate the circulation, breathing, digestion, excretion and the endocrine system. It is divided into two parts which act in different ways to balance each other.

The sympathetic division of the autonomic nervous system prepares the body for action by increasing the heart and respiration rate and increasing blood pressure. More blood will flow to the muscles and less to other areas, digestion is reduced, the skin will feel cold and damp and the muscles tense. This may be in response to pain or fear or feelings of stress. The parasympathetic division prepares the body for rest. It decreases heart rate and blood pressure and promotes digestion.

Massage, by its nature, should bring about relaxation and a reduction of stress. Stress is a necessary part of life which only becomes harmful when it is excessive or continuous to the point where it is difficult to cope with. Too much stress can bring about physical symptoms such as breathlessness, anxiety, tension headaches and insomnia. There are many relaxation techniques such as yoga and meditation taught to help to control the effects of stress and massage can be considered a very effective method of helping relaxation.

Aromatherapy massage is increasingly being used for clients who suffer from stress and stress related symptoms.

The essential oils of plants that are used in aromatherapy are all volatile and have their own distinctive smells. The receptors for the sense of smell, or olfaction, are in the lining of the upper part of the nose. Olfactory nerves carry messages from these cells to a specific part of the brain where the impulses are interpreted as odour and give rise to the sensation of smell. The sensation of smell happens quickly. Adaptation to odours also occurs quickly so that we become accustomed to most smells. (this accounts for failure to detect the smell of gas which accumulates slowly in a room). The sense of smell also 'tires' very quickly if it is exposed to too great a variety of smells one after the other.

The area of the brain where smell is registered is directly connected to a part of the base of the brain called the hypothalamus which is also connected to parts of the brain's limbic system, indeed it is often considered to be part of it. The limbic system includes areas of grey matter which control the emotional aspects of behaviour such as pain, pleasure, anger, rage and fear; also sorrow, sexual feelings, calmness and affection. The hypothalamus itself regulates other body activities through its control of the endocrine system and the autonomic nervous system. So in aromatherapy, for example, although essential oils affect the body by being absorbed into the blood stream, they can also affect the emotional responses by smell alone.

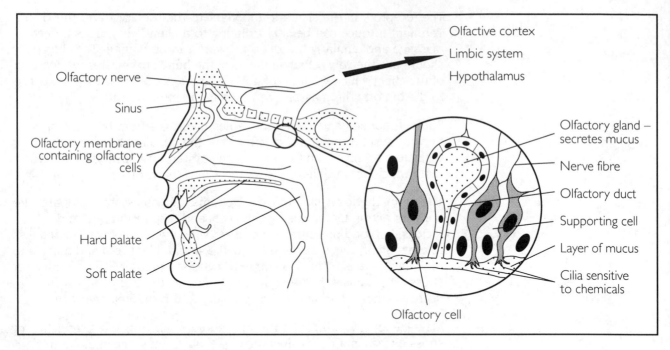

Figure 4.14 *The sense of smell (olfaction)*

KEY TERMS

You need to know what these words mean. Go back through the section or check in the glossary to find out.

Autonomic nervous system
Homeostasis
Limbic system

Receptors
Stimulus

Respiratory system

The respiratory system consists of the lungs and the tubes used for breathing.

Air can be taken in either by the mouth or the nose, however the functions of the nose are particularly important in breathing. The nose:

- warms the air as it enters the body
- moistens the air
- traps dust and dirt
- smells odours.

Air passes along the windpipe (trachea) and bronchi to the two lungs which occupy the major volume of the chest cavity with the heart between them. The lungs are divided into lobes. The windpipe divides

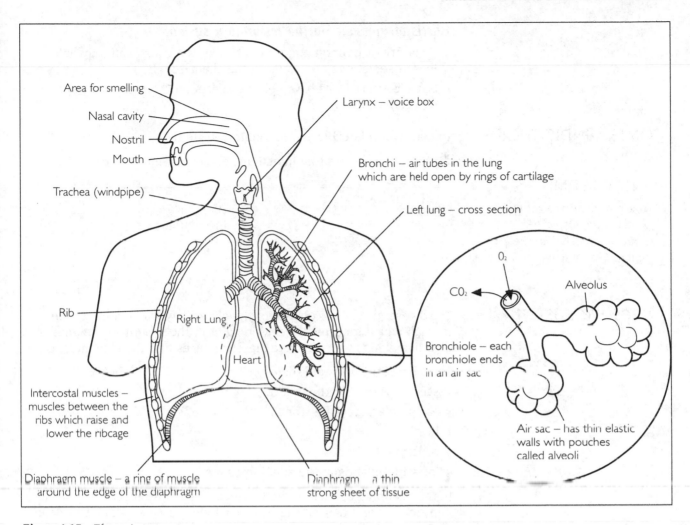

Figure 4.15 *The respiratory system*

into two bronchi, one to each lung, and the bronchi in turn divide into smaller and smaller tubes within the lung until the smallest, called bronchioles, end in air sacs called alveoli. The alveoli are bathed in blood and it is here that the exchange of gases between the air and the blood takes place, supplying the body with oxygen and removing carbon dioxide.

A normal rate of breathing in an adult is between 14 and 18 times a minute. This increases with exercise or during some illnesses.

Asthma

Asthma is a reaction, often allergic, characterised by attacks of wheezing and difficult breathing. As dust or other airborne substances may trigger an attack, care must be taken with asthmatic clients not to expose them to substances which are allergens. It is sometimes necessary to position a client to help breathing and an asthmatic will nearly always be more comfortable sitting up than lying down.

Effects of massage on the respiratory system

* Vibratory or pounding movements over the chest wall may help to loosen secretions and to make the client cough.
* Some essential oils have specific effects on the respiratory system especially when inhaled.

CONTRA-INDICATIONS to massage related to the respiratory system.

! Any acute respiratory infections, e.g. colds, flu, or bronchitis.

KEY TERMS

You need to know what these words mean. Go back through the section or check in the glossary to find out.

Allergens	Bronchi
Alveoli	Bronchioles

Digestive system

The digestive system consists of the alimentary canal, a long tube through which food passes extending from the mouth to the anus, and digestive glands which secrete digestive juices into the alimentary canal.

The digestive glands are the:

* salivary glands in the mouth
* gastric glands in the stomach
* liver
* pancreas
* intestinal glands in the small intestine.

In the oesophagus, before the food reaches the stomach, and in the intestines after it has left the stomach, food is pushed along by rhythmic contractions called peristalsis. During an abdominal massage movements are performed over the lower part of the stomach and over the large and small intestine. It is important to know the position of these parts of the system as they are not protected by the skeleton and will be vulnerable to pressure being put on them.

Effects of massage on the digestive system

* Gentle movements over the large intestine in a clockwise direction may stimulate peristalsis and prevent constipation.

CONTRA-INDICATIONS to massage related to the digestive system.

! Avoid the abdominal area after a heavy meal.

! Any pain in the abdomen.

KEY TERMS

You need to know what these words mean. Go back through the section or check in the glossary to find out.

Alimentary canal	Peristalsis

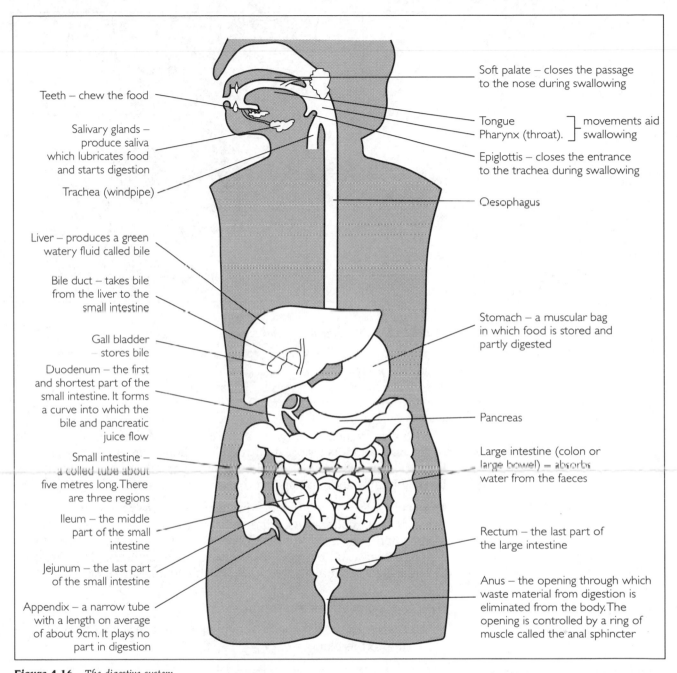

Teeth – chew the food

Salivary glands – produce saliva which lubricates food and starts digestion

Trachea (windpipe)

Liver – produces a green watery fluid called bile

Bile duct – takes bile from the liver to the small intestine

Gall bladder – stores bile

Duodenum – the first and shortest part of the small intestine. It forms a curve into which the bile and pancreatic juice flow

Small intestine – a coiled tube about five metres long. There are three regions

Ileum – the middle part of the small intestine

Jejunum – the last part of the small intestine

Appendix – a narrow tube with a length on average of about 9cm. It plays no part in digestion

Soft palate – closes the passage to the nose during swallowing

Tongue
Pharynx (throat).] movements aid swallowing

Epiglottis – closes the entrance to the trachea during swallowing

Oesophagus

Stomach – a muscular bag in which food is stored and partly digested

Pancreas

Large intestine (colon or large bowel) – absorbs water from the faeces

Rectum – the last part of the large intestine

Anus – the opening through which waste material from digestion is eliminated from the body. The opening is controlled by a ring of muscle called the anal sphincter

Figure 4.16 *The digestive system*

Renal system

The renal, or urinary, system consists of two kidneys, the tubes called ureters passing to the bladder, the bladder and the tube through which urine is expelled, the urethra.

Blood passes through the kidneys which remove unwanted substances from the blood and pass them in the form of urine to the bladder. When the pressure of urine in the bladder reaches a certain level it triggers a reflex to relax one of the muscles controlling the outlet. Another muscle is under voluntary control and can override the reflex to prevent urine being released until a convenient time.

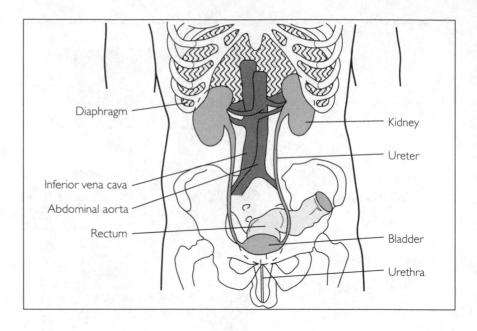

Figure 4.17 *The renal system (anterior view)*

The kidneys are delicate organs which are protected by the ribs, muscles of the back and a layer of fat surrounding them. However, pressure over them can be very uncomfortable and massage movements such as beating and pounding must not be used in the area.

The bladder is situated behind the pubic bone and when empty looks like a deflated balloon. As urine volume increases it becomes pear shaped and rises up into the abdominal cavity. During massage any pressure over a full bladder will be intensely uncomfortable, therefore always suggest that a client empties the bladder before a body massage.

Effects of massage on the renal system

* Stimulation of the lymphatic system may increase the amount of urine passing to the bladder.

CONTRA-INDICATIONS to massage related to the renal system.

! Over the abdomen in someone who has had a kidney transplant.

— KEY TERMS —

You need to know what these words mean. Go back through the section or check in the glossary to find out.	Reflex	Renal	Urinary

Endocrine system

The endocrine system is a control system of the body which works with the nervous system to maintain homeostasis. Homeostasis describes the state in which the body's internal environment stays constant. Whereas the nervous system controls the body by electrical impulses sent along nerves, the endocrine system works by releasing chemical messengers from endocrine glands into the blood stream. These are called hormones.

Endocrine gland	Hormone	Action of hormone
Pituitary gland	Growth hormone	Stimulates growth of bone and muscle
	Prolactin	Stimulates the breasts to produce milk in the female at the time of giving birth and afterwards maintains the milk supply
	Oxytocin	Stimulates the uterus in the female to contract at the end of pregnancy

The pituitary gland also produces hormones that control the function of all other endocrine glands

Hypothalamus	(Various)	Control the pituitary gland
Thyroid gland	Thyroid hormone	Controls metabolic rate
Parathyroid gland	Parathyroid hormone	Regulates the amount of calcium in the blood
Adrenal glands	Adrenaline	Prepares the body for physical action
	Corticosteroids	Help to maintain homeostasis
Pancreas	Insulin	Reduces the level of glucose (sugar) in the blood
	Glucagon	Raises the level of glucose in the blood
Testes	Androgens (male sex hormones)	Control the development and function of the male sex organs and control development of secondary sexual characteristics
Ovaries	Oestrogens (female sex hormones)	Control the development and function of the female sex organs and control development of secondary sexual characteristics
	Progesterone	Prepares for and maintains pregnancy

Table 4.3 *Endocrine glands and the hormones they produce*

The amount of hormone released by an endocrine gland is determined by the need for the hormone at any given time. The body is normally regulated so that there is no over or under-production of hormone. There are times when the regulating mechanism does not operate properly and hormonal levels are too high or too low. When this happens endocrine disorders result.

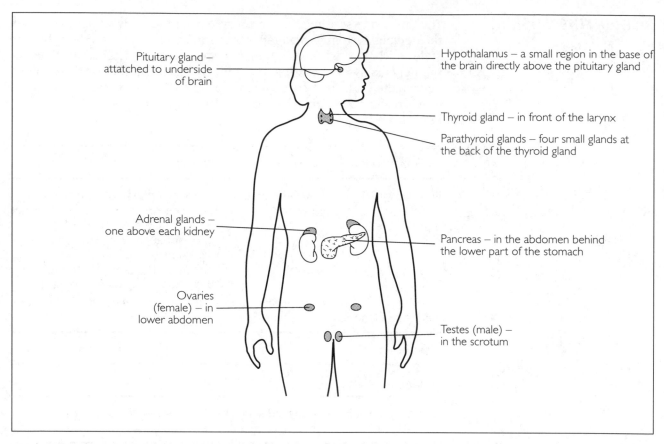

Figure 4.18   *The position of endocrine glands*

Some endocrine disorders which may be encountered by therapists are outlined below:

1 Hypothyroidism – too little output from the thyroid gland causes the body to retain water so that the face and body often look puffy, the skin looks thick and coarse and the hair is thin, dull and lifeless. Other symptoms may be lethargy and a tendency to gain weight. It is much more common in women than in men.

2 Hyperthyroidism – too much output from the thyroid gland, causing weight loss, anxiety, tremor in the hands, increased sweating and a fast pulse.

3 Diabetes – too little output of insulin from the pancreas, resulting in glucose building up in the blood. There are different types of diabetes which affect 1–2% of the population. People with diabetes may have related conditions such as high blood pressure, other circulatory troubles, altered sensation in the limbs, eyesight problems and poor healing of the skin, especially in the feet.

ACTIVITY

Carry out some research to find out about other disorders of the endocrine system, especially those which might alter a person's appearance in some way.

Effects of massage on the endocrine system

General massage, by combating stress, can support the endocrine system in maintaining homeostasis. Some essential oils used in aromatherapy have an effect on the system, either on the glands themselves or through the action of phytohormones (plant hormones) on the corresponding human hormones.

CONTRA-INDICATIONS

to massage related to the endocrine system.

! Care must be taken when using massage on areas of the body particularly affected by diabetes.

! Some essential oils are contra-indicated, particularly during pregnancy, due to their hormonal actions.

Stress

Massage and aromatherapy are recommended for-stress related conditions. Therefore it is important to have some idea of the nature of stress.

Stress is any stimulus which creates a disturbance in the body which upsets homeostasis. Stress may be caused by:

* heat or cold
* noise
* worry about work or relationships
* pain or illness.

Most stresses are mild and routine. The body has many regulating devices which combat routine stress and 'balance' the body again. Stress only becomes harmful when it is continuous, difficult to cope with and when it disrupts normal life. Whether stress becomes harmful depends on the person's ability to cope, the amount of stress involved and the length of time the stress continues.

Too much stress can cause a state of anxiety or depression and produce feelings of fear and anger. These may in turn cause physical symptoms in the body such as:

* headaches
* chest pain
* breathlessness
* skin rashes
* abdominal pain and indigestion
* irritability
* mood swings
* poor performance at work.

Stress over a long period of time results in general adaptation syndrome, a condition where temporary changes become chronic and the general level of health declines.

49

Illnesses which may be associated with stress are:

* cardiovascular disease
* respiratory disease
* cancer
* depression
* stomach ulcers.

Stress can also depress the body's immune system.

Immune system

The essential function of the immune system is defence against infection. Immunity of the body to attack is obtained when the body produces antibodies in response to antigens.

Antigens

Antigens are substances which stimulate the body to produce antibodies, e.g. bacteria, viruses, pollen and some foods

Antibodies

Antibodies are made by white blood cells called lymphocytes and are found in body tissues, blood and lymph nodes. They are proteins called immunoglobulins.

Immunity can:

* be total when all antigens are destroyed by antibodies
* be partial when the antigens cause some reaction in the body
* fail when the antigens are not destroyed and infection or reaction follows.

Autoimmune disease

Some diseases result when the immune system fails to function properly and the body produces antibodies which destroy its own cells. Examples of autoimmune diseases are some thyroid disease, rheumatoid arthritis and colitis.

Allergy is an overreaction of the body's immune system against a substance to which it has become sensitive.

ACTIVITY

By questioning family and friends find out how many of them have allergies and how they are affected by them.

People who have had an organ transplant such as a kidney or heart transplant have their immune system depressed by drugs to prevent the system from rejecting and destroying the new organ. Such people will have less resistance to infection.

Effects of massage on the immune system

Because of the calming effects of massage and its benefits in the treatment of stress, massage and aromatherapy are now thought to help to boost a depressed immune system. They are two of the complementary therapies being extensively used in diseases such as AIDS where the immune system is failing to cope with infection.

ACTIVITY

Find out which other complementary therapies are said to help stress-related conditions.

KEY TERMS

You need to know what these words mean. Go back through the section or look in the glossary to find out.

Antigens	Endocrine	Metabolic rate
Antibodies	Homeostasis	Phytohormones

5 Massage techniques

After working through this chapter you will be able to:

➤ explain the importance of continuity, rhythm and depth
➤ demonstrate suitable hand exercises for improving flexibility and strength
➤ obtain and react to client feedback
➤ demonstrate correct standing posture
➤ describe and demonstrate the five major categories of massage
➤ describe the uses, points of care and contra-indications specific to each category.

Massage is often called soft tissue manipulation. Soft tissue is a general term to cover all the superficial tissues other than bone, i.e. skin, fat, muscle and other connective tissue such as ligaments and tendons that may be affected by massage. While a knowledge of the structures of the body is important to develop and adapt massage, an in depth knowledge is not absolutely essential when starting to learn. Ideally the practical skills of massage and the theoretical knowledge of the structures and functions of the body should be studied together.

The hands are very sensitive and dextrous parts of the body so that while they are performing massage strokes they will also be receiving information about the body being worked on; information such as the temperature of the body, texture of the skin, firmness of the muscles, the relative thinness or fatness of the body and of course whether the hands are working over bony or soft tissue.

The sensitivity of the hands must be used to assess the state of the tissues and to learn about the client. It is a very direct form of feedback. If you cause pain or discomfort you should feel the client react and similarly if your touch is too light many people will respond by tensing the area. A question such as, 'Is that too deep?', will show that you are concentrating, thinking about the massage and are willing to adapt it to the individual client. This is a very important part of the caring process which enhances the client–therapist relationship.

Whenever possible position yourself so that you can see the client's face to observe any reactions. Eventually, the adaptation of massage to the individual should become intuitive and almost automatic but never uncaring.

> **REMEMBER**
>
> *It is easy to let your mind wander when massaging. The moment this happens the massage will suffer. Always concentrate on what you are doing.*

There are three particularly important constituents of a good massage which should always be kept in mind.

* Continuity.
* Rhythm.
* Depth.

Continuity

Interruptions in the massage routine should be kept to a minimum with the hands staying in contact as much as possible and the transition from one stroke to another made without a break. This achieves continuity.

Rhythm

The rhythm should be even and steady with no jerkiness that would disturb the routine. The rate may be slow for relaxation or faster for more stimulation. Some therapists find music a help to set a mood but care must be taken not to try to fit the movements to the music. (Care should also be taken to check that the choice of music does not irritate the client.)

Depth

The depth of massage should be appropriate to the needs and physical state of the client. Thus the depth of massage used for a young, fit person would be different from that used on someone who was elderly and frail. However, it should be remembered that most people prefer a firm massage and that in the initial treatment the client's reactions and opinions should be sought and recorded for future reference. The depth of the massage is altered by using the weight of your body effectively, so the posture and stance of the therapist is of vital importance in performing effective massage.

GOOD PRACTICE ▷ **Stance**

The therapist must be able to carry out any of the massage movements along the whole length of the part of the body being treated without strain. This can be achieved by taking up an effective working position and maintaining good posture. The feet should always be apart to provide a good base and help balance while working. The line between the feet should be in the same direction as the direction of movement. This enables the whole body to be moved in the direction of the movement with the weight being transferred from one foot to the other. In the main, the feet should be in either the walk-standing position with one foot in front of the other or in stride-standing with the feet level but apart. The back should always be straight to reduce strain and the shoulders relaxed. The knees may be bent to reduce height instead of bending the back. Try to keep the arms out away from the body to help attain a relaxed movement.

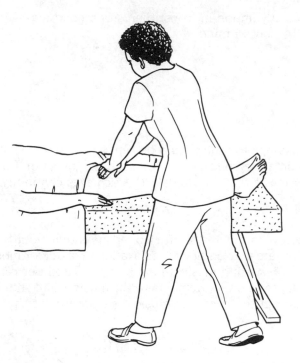

Figure 5.1 *Walk-standing: correct*

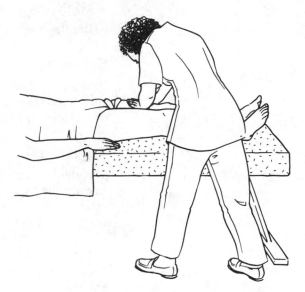

Figure 5.2 *Walk-standing: incorrect*

Hands

Hands must be relaxed and warm. Tension in the hands is soon detected by the client and can be very uncomfortable. The hands will be fully in contact with the body for the majority of the massage and need to be strong and flexible as well as being sensitive enough to assess the state of the tissues being worked on. The more massage is practised, the stronger and more flexible the hands become.

There are many simple exercises which can be carried out daily to help to mobilise and strengthen the hands and wrists. One such sequence of simple hand exercises is described below.

1 Hold the hands at chest level and shake them loosely and vigorously for a count of ten.

2 Touch the fingertips of one hand to the fingertips of the other and press so that the fingers and thumbs are widespread and pushed back. Bounce the fingers together to increase the range of movement in the fingers.

3 Place the palms of the hands together and lift the elbows so that the wrists are bent at right angles and press one hand against the other alternately back and forth to mobilise the wrists.

4 Lightly clench the hands at chest level and rotate the hands ten times in one direction, then ten times in the other direction.

5 Clench and unclench the hands very quickly about ten times and then repeat the fist shaking exercise.

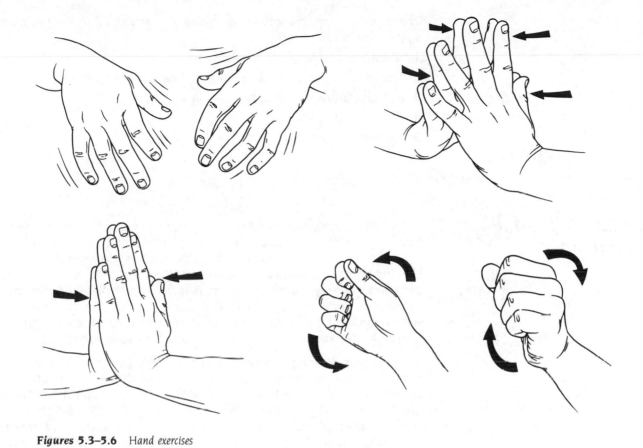

Figures 5.3–5.6 Hand exercises

Lubricant

Most therapists use some form of lubricant on the hands to prevent the hands dragging on the skin. Whatever lubricant is chosen, there should never be more than the minimum used; just enough to prevent dragging, but not enough to make the hands slip and slide with loss of control. More lubricant can be added during the massage if needed, but having to remove excess is disruptive. The choice of lubricant is made between a cream, an oil or talcum powder and is discussed in Chapter 2, *The working environment*.

If you need to add oil during the massage, dribble a little onto the back of the hand which is on the body, then pick the oil up by passing the other hand over it.

GOOD PRACTICE ▷ *Before you start a massage:*

* *make sure you have all the necessary equipment within reach*
* *check that everything is clean and hygienic*
* *warm and exercise your hands if necessary*
* *wash your hands.*

The massage movements in this chapter are described in the traditional way in the following groups.

1 Effleurage and stroking.

2 Petrissage – to include kneading, picking up, wringing and rolling.

3 Tapotement (also called percussion).

4 Vibrations and shaking.

5 Friction and frictions.

Effleurage and stroking

The word effleurage means 'to stroke', but the two terms have come to have slightly different meanings in massage today. In both movements the hands move over the skin in the same manner. However they differ in the direction of movement. In effleurage the movement is in the direction of the lymphatic and venous flow and so will affect the flow of blood and lymph in the vessels. Stroking is used to describe similar movements but direction is not important and rather than affecting the flow of blood and lymph it is mainly used for its sensory effects.

The rhythmic, flowing movements of effleurage and stroking are most important in a general massage. As they cover the whole area to be treated these movements will be used to start and finish the massage, spread the chosen lubricant, link other strokes together and even to fill in a gap when you can't think what to do next! The speed and depth of the strokes in effleurage and stroking may be altered according to the effects desired. Slow deep strokes are relaxing while brisker, more superficial strokes tend to be stimulating.

Effleurage

Stance   Walk-standing in the direction that the hands will move.

Hands   One hand or two may be used depending on the size of the part to be treated. If one hand only is working, then the other can be used to support the part. Usually the whole surface of the palm and fingers is used but on very small areas, the padded surface of the fingers and thumb may be used.

The hands and fingers should be relaxed and fit to the part so that they are in perfect contact with the skin. If any part of the hand is held stiffly then the effleurage strokes will feel hard and uncomfortable. To begin a stroke the hands are placed on the end of the part of the body furthest away from the heart, the distal extremity, e.g. on the foot to begin effleurage to the leg or on the lower back at the start of effleurage to the back. The fingers should be pointing in the direction of movement. They are moved firmly upwards over the skin to cover the required area and then brought more lightly back down to the starting point.

REMEMBER

Physiological effects of massage are described in the previous chapter.

Uses

* To start and finish massage to an area.
* To link between other strokes.
* To accustom the client to the therapist's touch.
* To spread the lubricant evenly.
* To warm the skin and produce an erythema.
* To induce relaxation and reduce muscle tone.
* To improve lymphatic and venous drainage.
* To remove dead skin cells, stimulate sweat and sebaceous glands, and improve the suppleness of the skin.

Stroking

Stance   Walk-standing as for effleurage.

Hands   Relaxed, moulded to the part and in full contact with the skin. The strokes may be in any direction over the skin, e.g. downward as in returning from an effleurage movement on the back or leg, circular as in circling around the scapulae on the upper back or sideways as may be done at the waist. The depth and speed will vary according to the intensity of the effects required and occasionally one hand may be placed over the other to increase the depth, this is called reinforced stroking.

Uses

* To act as a link between other movements.
* To get the hands to a new position without breaking the continuity of the massage.
* To warm the area and produce an erythema.
* To aid relaxation and reduce muscle tone.
* To remove dead skin cells, stimulate sweat and sebaceous glands and improve the suppleness of the skin.

SAFE PRACTICE ▷ *Points of care for effleurage and stroking*

* *Don't drag on the skin.*
* *Use more lubricant on hairy skin and whenever possible work with the natural lie of the hair. On very hairy skin omit effleurage completely.*
* *Lighten the pressure as the hands pass over bony or sensitive areas.*

CONTRA-INDICATIONS   to effleurage and stroking.

❗ Over any areas of skin showing signs of infection or skin conditions which may spread.

❗ Over any bruised area.

<table>
<tr><td>

REMEMBER

Advice on medical referral is given in Chapter 3 – Consultation.

</td></tr>
</table>

! Over obvious varicose veins which are painful or tender to the touch. Light strokes may be used over superficial veins that are not tender.

! Over an area where there has been a deep venous thrombosis or thrombo phlebitis.

PROGRESS CHECK Try the following practical exercises. (Note: the term client is used throughout even though it is presumed that practice will take place on a colleague or other model.)

---

1 Effleurage to the back

With a client lying prone on a couch of suitable height, cover the legs and buttocks so that the length of the back is exposed. The client's arms may be loosely by the side or bent up with the hands beside the head.

Stance   By the side of the couch in walk-standing at the level of the client's hips so that you can reach the whole length of the back from the base of the spine to the neck. Your feet should be pointing towards the head of the couch.

Hands   Relaxed and warm with a little of the oil or other lubricant spread on them. Place both hands on the lower back with fingers pointing up the back with the whole of the hands in contact. Now move both hands up the back one on each side of the spine to the top of the back where the fingers will curl over the top of the shoulders. In order to reach the shoulders and keep the depth of the stroke even you must move your body weight from the back foot to the front foot, bending the front knee slightly.

Keeping contact, bring the hands back down to the base of the spine. The downward stroke should be lighter and more superficial than the upward stroke and be a little further out to the side. Repeat this movement a number of times until a rhythm is built up. Increase the depth on the upward effleurage movement but keep the speed steady and even. Move your weight from the back foot to the front foot in the upward movement, and use your body weight to apply pressure.

SAFE PRACTICE ▷ *Keep your back straight to avoid back strain.*

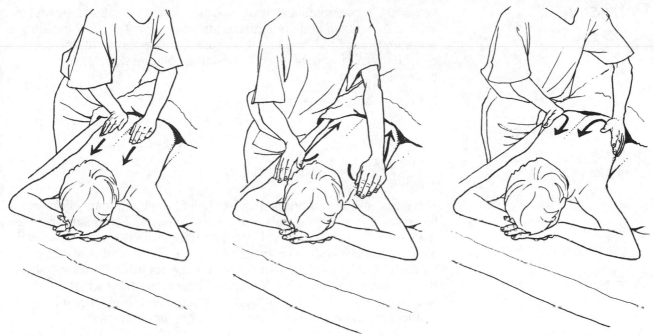

Figure 5.7 *Effleurage to the back*

2 *Reinforced stroking*

The client should be lying prone with the back exposed.

Stance Walk-standing at waist level facing the head of the couch.

Hands Make sure there is enough lubricant on the hands and place them between the scapulae with one hand over the other. Move both hands upwards between the bones, around one scapula and then the other in a figure of eight pattern. The pressure should be deeper on the upward movement and there should be no pressure at all as the hands cross the bony points of the spine.

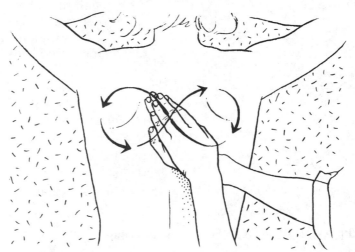

Figure 5.8 *Reinforced stroking to the back*

REMEMBER

Keep the speed steady and even. Transfer body weight and maintain good posture.

Petrissage

Petrissage movements are those in which soft tissues are compressed against underlying bone or squeezed in some way. The term kneading is sometimes used to describe all petrissage movements, but more correctly should only be used to describe compression against underlying bone.

Petrissage movements include:

* kneading
* picking up
* wringing
* rolling.

These squeezing, compressing movements have a pumping effect on the blood and lymphatic vessels in the soft tissues and stimulate the drainage of lymph and blood. Many of the petrissage movements will also put a slight stretch on the tissue, helping to maintain elasticity and mobility. This is particularly relevant for the superficial muscles where the massage may stretch the muscle fibres along their length as in wringing or across their width as in rolling. The movements will cause dilation of superficial blood vessels causing an erythema.

Kneading

Kneading is a circular movement where the hand moves the skin on the deeper tissues. The hands do not move over the skin except to move to the next part to be treated.

Stance   Walk-standing in the direction of the main movement.

Hands   Depending on the size of the area being treated kneading can be performed with both hands at a time, or with one hand, or with a smaller part of the hand, such as the palm or the thumbs. The pressure is varied with greater pressure being applied on the upward part of the circle. The pressure is increased by the use of body weight. Both hands may be used together or alternately, or a single hand may be used with the other supporting the part. Where the tissues are dense and thick, one hand may be placed over the other to give extra force and depth to the movement, often called reinforced kneading.

Uses

* To stimulate lymphatic drainage in the muscles and other tissues.
* To stimulate the supply of arterial blood in the muscles and other tissues.
* To produce dilation of the superficial blood vessels (vaso-dilation) and erythema.
* To mobilise subcutaneous tissue.

CONTRA-INDICATIONS   to kneading.

! Over bruised or tender areas.

60

SAFE PRACTICE ▷ Points of care for kneading

* There is a tendency when kneading to use the 'heel' of the hand to exert pressure. This should be avoided as it can cause acute discomfort to the client.
* Avoid pressure over bony points.
* Don't drag on the skin.

PROGRESS CHECK   Try the following practical exercises.

1 Single-handed kneading to the thigh

The client should be lying supine with the leg nearest you uncovered.

Stance Walk-standing facing the head of the couch at knee level.

Hands A minimum amount of oil should be used as the hands must not slide on the skin. Place one hand on the inner surface of the knee for support. The other hand is placed on the outer surface of the upper thigh with the arm and elbow held well away from the side – this is the working hand. The outer, working, hand is moved in a circular fashion on the outer thigh moving the skin over the deeper tissues. The circle should be made three or four times, then the hand should slide down the thigh a little and the circles repeated until the hand reaches to just above the knee. The movement can be repeated by sliding the hand up the outer thigh to the starting point. The outer hand then becomes the supporting hand while the inner hand repeats the movement down the inner thigh to the knee. Pressure will be lighter on the inside of the leg as the tissue is more sensitive.

REMEMBER

Pass lightly over bony points such as the greater trochanter of the femur. Apply counter-pressure with the non-working hand.

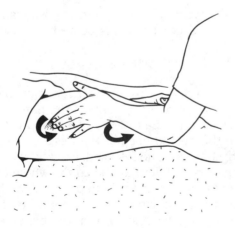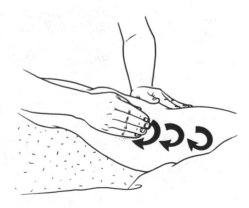

Figure 5.9 *Single-handed kneading*

2 Double-handed kneading

Stance   As for single-handed kneading.

Hands   One on the inside and one on the outside of the upper thigh – now both are working hands. The elbows should be bent and away from the sides so that the thigh is squeezed between both hands. The hands are moved alternately in a circular fashion, maintaining the squeezing effect and only moving over the skin to progress gradually down the leg to the knee. When the knee is reached both the hands slide up the thigh to the starting position and the movement is repeated. This is quite hard work and needs practice to be able to do it without strain.

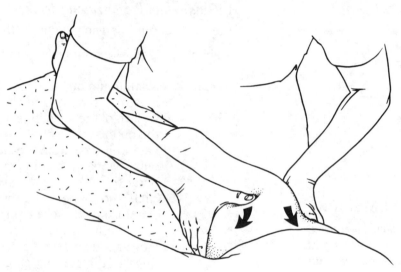

REMEMBER

Don't hold your breath while working.

Figure 5.10   *Double-handed kneading*

Picking up

Picking up is a petrissage movement where the soft tissue is picked up, lifted away from the deeper tissue or bone, squeezed and released.

Stance   Walk-standing in the direction of movement.

Hands   One hand or two may be used but it is easier to start with one hand, using the other to support the part. In single-handed picking up the part of the hand used is the V between the thumb and fingers. The tissues being worked on are lifted, squeezed and released. Be careful not to dig in with the fingers and thumb and keep the whole of the V as well as the palm in contact to avoid pinching. At the start of the movement apply compression through the hand, then grasp the tissue and lift it away from the bone before releasing it and moving on.

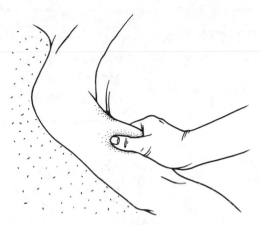

Figure 5.11 *Single-handed picking up*

Double-handed picking up is used on large muscular areas such as the front of the thigh where both hands are needed to span the muscle. The hands are arranged so that the thumb of one hand lies alongside the index finger of the other forming a much wider V-shape with which to grasp the muscle. The action is the same – press, squeeze, lift, release, and move on. The whole of the palms of the hands should be in contact.

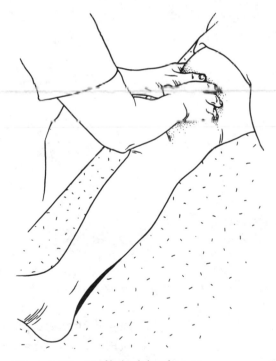

Figure 5.12 *Double handed picking up*

Uses

* To stimulate venous and lymphatic flow.
* To stimulate arterial flow.
* To loosen tight subcutaneous tissue.

SAFE PRACTICE ▷ *Points of care for picking up*
  * *Keep palms in contact.*
  * *Don't dig fingers in.*
  * *Keep shoulders relaxed.*

CONTRA-INDICATIONS   to picking up.

! Over bruised or tender tissue.

PROGRESS CHECK   Try the following practical exercises.

1 Single-handed picking up

On your own forearm, grasp the muscles on the thumb side of your forearm just below elbow level with the palm of the other hand so that the muscles fit into the V between thumb and forefinger. Lift the muscles away from the bone, squeeze, release and slide the hand a little lower and repeat the movement until you reach just above the wrist. Slide the hand back up to the elbow and repeat.

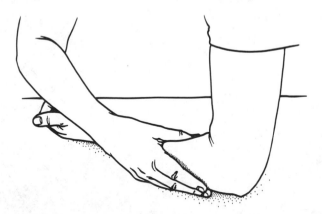

Figure 5.13 *Practising single-handed picking up*

2 Double-handed picking up on the front of the thigh

The client should be supine lying with one leg uncovered.

Stance   Walk-standing at knee level.

Hands   Place both hands on the front of the thigh with one hand overlapping the other as described. The V of the hands should be as wide as possible. With both hands, press down, grasp the large quadriceps muscle mass between the hands, lift away from the bone and gently release the pressure. Slide the hands a little lower down and repeat until you can feel that there is no more muscle mass just above the knee. To reach the top of the thigh again the hands can slide up or can repeat the picking up with the hands moving upward.

Wringing

Wringing is a petrissage movement similar to picking up. The tissues are compressed and picked up from the bone as in picking up, but instead of then being released they are passed from hand to hand in a wringing movement.

Stance Stride-standing or walk-standing facing across the area to be treated.

Hands Wringing is always performed with both hands. They are placed on the part with the fingers on one side and the thumbs on the other. The arms must be held well out to the sides with the elbows half bent. Muscle and superficial tissue is compressed and scooped up between the fingers and thumb of each hand, then the fingers of one hand pull the tissue towards you while the thumb of the other hand pushes it away. The hands move along the length of the muscle, wringing as they go. The smaller the muscle is that is being worked on the more the fingers are used rather than the whole hand, e.g. across the shoulders where there is no room for the whole hand.

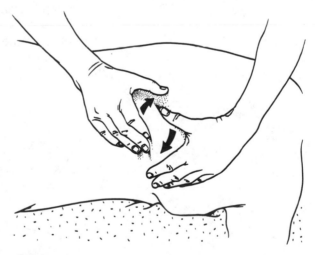

Figure 5.14 *Wringing on superficial tissues*

Uses

- To improve elasticity by stretching along the length of muscle.
- To soften hard, subcutaneous fatty tissue.
- To improve local circulation.

65

SAFE PRACTICE ▷ *Points of care for wringing*

* *Don't twist the hands on the skin as this can be painful.*
* *Keep fingers and thumbs straight so that the tips don't dig in.*

CONTRA-INDICATIONS to wringing.

! Bruised or tender tissue.

! Areas of stretched skin.

! Areas of poor muscle tone, e.g. on an older client.

PROGRESS CHECK Try the following practical exercises.

Wringing to the muscles of the thigh

Stance   Stride-standing facing across the client.

Hands   Both on the upper inner thigh with fingers together and thumbs wide apart. Pick up the muscle with one hand then the other and start wringing by pulling with the fingers of one hand and at the same time pushing away with the thumb of the other hand. The movement is reversed so that the muscle is kept lifted away from the bone and is passed from hand to hand. Move the hands down the inner thigh, up the front of the thigh and down the outer surface wringing all the time. To reach the outer surface you must bend your knees to get your height down to the necessary level.

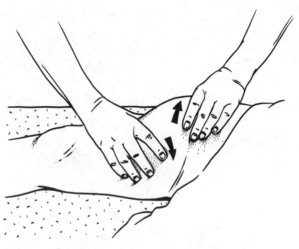

Figure 5.15 *Wringing to the muscles of the thigh*

Wringing to the shoulders

The client must be lying prone with the upper back exposed.

Stance Walk-standing facing the head of the couch.

Hands Cupped over the shoulder furthest away from you. Pick up the muscle at the top of the shoulder between the fingers and thumb of both hands and wring the muscle by pulling with the fingers of one hand and pushing with the thumb of the other. Move the hands across the shoulder towards the neck. When the neck is reached keep one hand in contact while the other moves across to the other shoulder. Follow with the other hand and continue wringing across to the point of the near shoulder. This can be repeated back and forth across the tops of the shoulders.

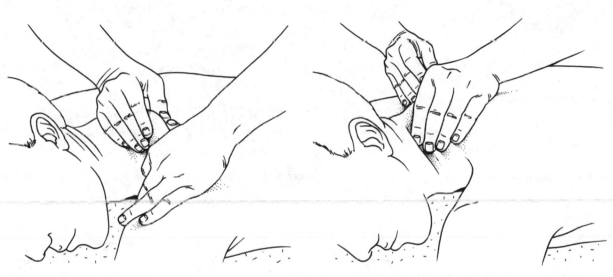

Figure 5.16 *Wringing to the shoulders*

Rolling

The most common type of rolling is skin rolling where the skin and subcutaneous tissue is rolled between fingers and thumb. Muscle rolling can be performed as a deeper form of the movement across muscle fibres.

Skin rolling

Stance Facing across the part to be treated with the feet in walk or stride-standing.

Hands Placed flat on the part with the thumbs spread wide and their tips touching.

The fingers pull the tissue up into a roll against the thumbs which then push the roll of skin back towards the fingers.

Keep a steady rhythm as the hands move up and down the area to be treated. This movement is easy when performed on the opposite side of the body from the therapist, i.e. pushing the roll of skin away with the thumbs but is more difficult when being performed on the side nearest the therapist. Here the therapist can either twist the upper body and arms so that the movement can be carried out as before or reverse the hand movement so that the fingers push a roll of skin towards the thumbs.

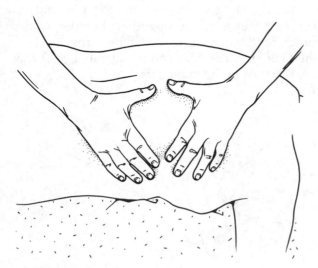

Figure 5.17   *Skin rolling – hand position*

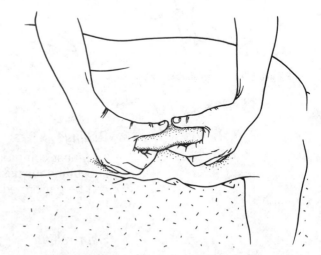

Figure 5.18   *Skin rolling – pulling the tissue into a roll with the fingers*

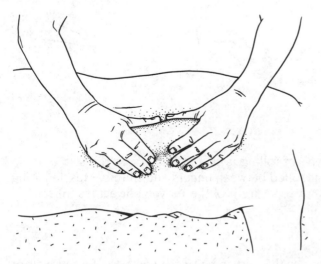

Figure 5.19   *Skin rolling – squeeze and lift*

Figure 5.20   *Skin rolling – pushing the roll back with the thumbs*

Uses

- To stimulate the circulation in the skin.
- To soften hard subcutaneous tissue such as fat.
- To induce relaxation by the rhythmic nature of the strokes.

* To improve elasticity of the skin.
* To soften an area around old scar tissue.

Points of care for skin rolling

* *Don't allow the fingers and thumb to pinch the skin.*
* *Be prepared for some clients to find this ticklish over the ribs.*
* *Only turn your body and arms to work on the near side if you can do it without strain on your back.*

CONTRA-INDICATIONS

to skin rolling.

! Over an area of stretched or loose skin.

! Over bruised or tender skin.

PROGRESS CHECK

Try the following practical exercise.

Skin rolling to the back

The client should be lying prone with the back exposed.

Stance Walk-standing facing across client just above waist level.

Hands Placed on the side of the back away from you at the client's waist. The fingers should be straight with the thumbs as far away from the forefinger as possible. The tips of the thumbs should be touching and those of the forefingers almost touching. With the flat of the hand in contact with the skin, pull the fingers towards you so that the skin moves with them, press down with your thumbs and push the resulting roll of skin towards the fingers with the long surface of the thumbs. Repeat the movement in a smooth rhythm up and down the side of the body.

> **REMEMBER**
>
> *Keep your back straight — bend your knees to reduce your height.*

Muscle rolling

This is similar to skin rolling but is deeper and works across the fibres of a muscle.

Stance The same as for skin rolling.

Hands Placed in a similar position as for skin rolling but over a suitable muscle. The fingers and thumbs are pressed down so that the muscle bulges between them. The thumbs are rolled towards the fingers across the muscle fibres or slightly along them, whichever is most comfortable for the client.

Uses

* To relieve tension and adhesions in the muscle.
* To improve circulation in the muscle.

Points of care and contra-indications for muscle rolling are the same as for skin rolling.

Muscle rolling to the erector spinae

The client should be lying prone with the back uncovered.

Stance	Walk-standing facing across the client at chest level.
Hands	Place the hands flat on the far side of the back with the thumbs lying in the groove between the spine and the long muscle of the back (erector spinae). With the fingers feel for the far boundary of the muscle. Press firmly with the thumbs and fingers so that the muscle bulges between them and push across the muscle with the thumbs. Repeat down the length of the muscle to the base of the spine. To perform this movement on the side nearest you, you have to move the fingers towards the thumbs or work from the opposite side of the body.

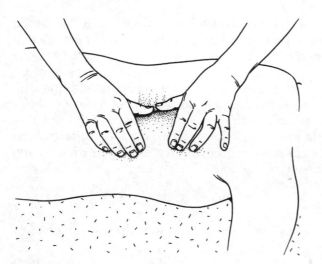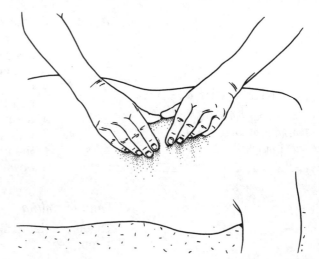

Figure 5.21   *Muscle rolling*

Tapotement/ percussion

The terms tapotement and percussion are interchangeable and, as the names suggest, describe a group of movements where the parts are struck repeatedly with soft blows of the hands. Both hands are usually used and they strike the part alternately. The movements must be light and bouncy, not heavy and solid. Practice is needed to achieve this and to acquire an easy, non-tiring rhythm. The wrists must be loose and the arms relaxed. There is always a tendency to hunch your shoulders and hold your breath when trying these movements.

All the movements are stimulating and are usually omitted from a relaxing style of massage.

Tapotement/percussion movements are:

* Hacking.
* Pounding.
* Clapping.
* Beating.

The easiest way to practise all percussion movements is on a pillow or cushion placed on the treatment couch. This allows you to adjust the depth and rhythm until you feel confident enough to try them on a client.

Hacking

Stance   Walk-standing, facing across the part to be treated.

Hands   Hacking is performed with a small part of the ulnar (little finger) side of the hands and the back of the little, ring and middle fingers. The elbows are bent and held well away from the body and the wrists are bent back as far as possible. The fingers should be loose, slightly apart and a little bent.

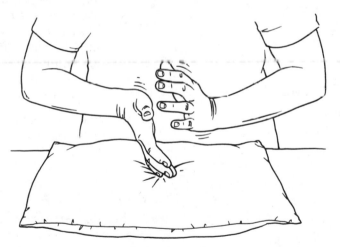

Figure 5.22   *Practising hacking on a pillow*

The movement is produced by rapidly striking the part with alternate hands. Only the forearms and wrists move, not the shoulders or elbows. It should be rapid and light making a tapping sound. On more muscular areas it can be a little slower and deeper.

Uses

* To stimulate superficial circulation and produce an erythema.
* To stimulate superficial muscle by producing a reflex contraction.

71

CONTRA-INDICATIONS

to hacking.

! Over any bruised or sensitive area.

! Over varicose veins.

PROGRESS CHECK Try the following practical exercise.

Hacking

With a pillow on the couch.

Stance	Stride-standing facing the couch.
Hands	Rest the ulnar (little finger) side of the hands on the pillow with the palms facing each other, the hands relaxed and only a little way apart. Bend the elbows to a right angle and take them away from your body. The wrists now should be fully extended. Keeping the elbows still, strike the pillow with alternate hands. Only the sides and backs of the little, ring and middle fingers and a small part of the side of the hand should strike the pillow. The striking should be so light as to almost flick the pillow rather than hit it.

When you have a steady rhythm move the hands to cover the whole surface of the pillow and try to vary the speed and depth.

REMEMBER

Don't hold your breath while working.

Pounding

This is a heavier percussion movement than hacking and should only be used over large, well-covered areas such as the gluteal region.

Stance	The same as for hacking.
Hands	The elbows and arms are held in the same position as for hacking but the hands should be loosely clenched so that a soft fist is made. The movement made is similar to hacking, using alternate hands to strike the part with the side of the loose fist.

Uses

- ⊛ To increase local circulation.
- ⊛ To soften fatty tissue.

CONTRA-INDICATIONS   to pounding.

! Over bony areas or on very thin clients.

! Over weak or poorly toned muscles.

! Over bruising or varicose veins.

PROGRESS CHECK   Try the following exercise.

Pounding

Using a pillow, with loosely clenched fists perform the same movement as for hacking.

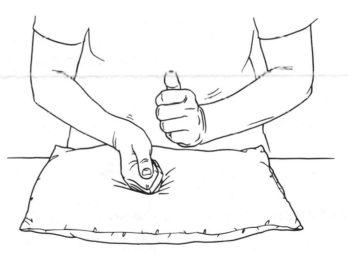

Figure 5.23 *Practising pounding on a pillow*

Clapping

Clapping is a percussion movement in which the area is struck with the hands cupped.

Stance   Face across the part to be treated with the feet in walk or stride-standing.

Hands   Although the palms of the hands are used to perform this movement, the hands should be cupped so that the centre of the palm does not touch the part. The fingers are held straight with the thumbs held close to the index fingers. The arms are held away from the sides of the body to allow for some movement at the elbows although most of the movement takes place at the wrists. The hands strike the part alternately and should produce a dull, hollow sound, not a slapping noise.

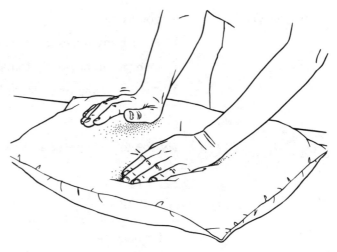

Figure 5.24 *Practising clapping on a pillow*

Uses

* To stimulate skin circulation.
* To shake deeper tissues and stimulate circulation.

SAFE PRACTICE ▷ *Points of care for clapping*
   * *Over sensitive skin the movement may be performed over a towel or blanket.*

CONTRA-INDICATIONS   to clapping.

❗ Over bruised or tender skin.

PROGRESS CHECK   Try the following exercise.

Clapping

Stance   Walk or stride-standing facing the pillow on the couch.

Hands   Place both hands palm down on the pillow and draw up the centre of the hand until middle of the palm is off the pillow. Start to strike the pillow with alternate hands, moving along the length of the pillow, with the hands staying quite close to each other.

— REMEMBER —
If you lose the rhythm of the strokes, change to another stroke for a while then try again.

74

Beating

Beating is a percussion movement performed as in clapping, but with the hands held in loose fists.

Stance   Facing across the part to be treated with the feet in walk or stride-standing.

Hands   Held in loose fists but with the ends of the fingers held straight instead of tucked into the fist (this provides the flat surface to strike the part). The thumbs are kept close to the side of the fist and the wrists kept very loose.

                 The therapist's arms are lifted so that the wrists droop then the part is struck with alternate fists. This may be changed to clapping by just opening and cupping the hand. The arm movement remains the same.

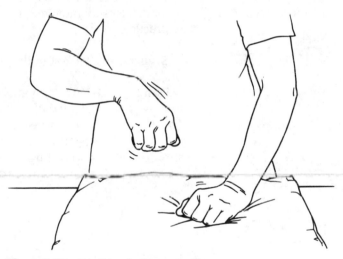

Figure 5.25   *Practising beating on a pillow*

Uses

* To soften hard, fatty tissue.

SAFE PRACTICE ▷ *Points of care for beating*
* *Only use over well-covered areas such as the gluteals.*

CONTRA-INDICATIONS   to beating.

!   Over bruised or tender areas.

!   Over weak muscles.

Beating

Repeat the exercise given for clapping but with the hand loosely clenched and the fingers straight

Vibrations and shaking

These types of movement involve producing a tremor or shake in the tissues. However, the techniques they employ and their uses are very different.

Vibrations

In the vibrations movement the effects are produced by the therapist vibrating the hands or fingers so that the vibrations are transmitted to the part being treated. The tremor may be produced by an up and down or side to side movement. It is difficult to do well and takes considerable practice.

Stance   Walk-standing facing across or along the part.

Hands   Only one hand works while the other supports the part. The arm is held outstretched and the hand placed firmly on the part. Either the whole hand, with fingers and thumb close together, or the tips of the fingers may be used. The hand and/or fingers are vibrated up and down or vibrated sideways to produce a fine tremor in the tissue, the hand always keeping contact with the skin.

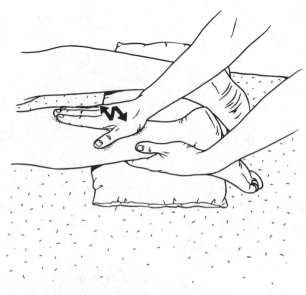

Figure 5.26   *Vibrations*

76

Uses

* Over the course of a nerve as a soothing mechanism.
* Over an area needing stimulation of lymphatic drainage.

SAFE PRACTICE ▷ *Points of care for vibrations*

* *Don't dig in with the finger tips.*

CONTRA-INDICATIONS   to vibrations.

! Over very poorly-covered areas.

PROGRESS CHECK   Try the following exercise.

Vibrations to the back of the thigh

The client should be lying prone with the back of one leg exposed.

Stance   Walk-standing facing the head of the couch at knee level.

Hands   Place the working hand flat, high up in the centre of the back of the thigh. The other hand rests on the side of the thigh to support it. Keeping the working arm outstretched, vibrate the hand up and down quite quickly and at the same time slide the hand down the centre of the back of the thigh to the level of the knee.

Shaking

This is a less fine movement than vibrations. The muscle area being treated is grasped by the hand or fingers, usually towards the origin or

REMEMBER

It helps the therapist to relax the shoulders occasionally while working. Do this by pushing them down to stretch the neck and then letting them spring back.

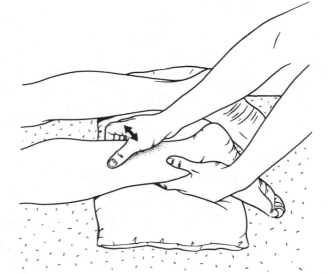

Figure 5.27 *Shaking*

insertion of the muscle, and then loosely shaken from side to side. In sports massage, and sometimes shiatsu treatments, the whole limb may be shaken by grasping the hand or foot and shaking the whole arm or leg sideways or up and down.

Uses

* To relax the muscles.

SAFE PRACTICE ▷ *Points of care for shaking*
* *Keep fingers as straight as possible to avoid digging in with the fingers.*

CONTRA-INDICATIONS

to shaking.

! Over thin or over-stretched muscles.

Friction and frictions

Although the names of the friction and frictions movements sound almost the same, they are completely different and are described together here in order to stress the differences. Friction is the fast rubbing of the skin, often used to warm the skin, whilst frictions are small deep movements on localised areas which move superficial tissues on deep ones. Friction may be described as a fast stroking movement and frictions as deep petrissage.

Friction

Stance   Walk or stride-standing facing in the direction of general movement.

Hands   The flat, palmar surface of hands and fingers are used with the hands held stiffly so that the palm and fingers are firm. The hands are rubbed quickly over the skin in any direction.

Uses

* To stimulate the local blood supply.
* To warm the area being treated.

SAFE PRACTICE ▷ *Points of care for friction*
* *Avoid any area with prominent moles or skin tags.*
* *Don't use in a relaxing-type massage without warning the client.*
* *If the skin is loose, only use very light pressure.*

CONTRA-INDICATIONS   to friction.

! Over very sensitive skin.

! Over very hairy skin.

PROGRESS CHECK   Try the following exercise.

Friction to the back
The client should be lying prone with the back uncovered.

Stance   Walk-standing facing the head of the couch at waist level.

Hands   Place flat on the back and hold stiff and firm, then, moving the hands briskly, rub the surface of the whole back in short random movements.

Frictions
Stance   Walk or stride-standing, close to the couch so that you are able to exert enough force.

Hands   The fingertips are used to apply frictions and the fingers must be held stiffly. The fingertips press firmly and move in small circles, with no sliding, over the skin. To move on lift the fingers, move to the next area, and continue. Small to and fro frictions are sometimes applied across particular muscle fibres. In each case superficial tissue is compressed and moved over the deeper tissues.

Uses
* To produce a localised erythema.
* To soften and stretch tight tissue such as scar tissue or adhesions in muscle.
* To ease the condition known as fibrositis which can be felt as hard bands of muscle fibres, especially in the upper back.
* To stimulate the spinal nerves when used down the sides of the spine.
* In sports massage over ligaments.

SAFE PRACTICE ▷ *Points of care for frictions*
* *Start the frictions fairly superficially and gradually increase the depth.*
* *Don't let your fingers bend back when applying pressure.*
* *Intersperse the frictions with effleurage movements to reduce discomfort.*
* *Areas of 'fibrositis' are tender, so be aware of the client's reactions.*
* *Always completely remove the fingers from the skin to progress to another area.*

CONTRA-INDICATIONS

to frictions.

❗ Over painful areas.

❗ Over bony points.

❗ Over any area of inflammation.

PROGRESS CHECK   Try the following exercise.

Frictions to the back

The client should be lying prone with the back uncovered.

Stance   Walk-standing close to the couch at waist level.

Hands   Place the middle finger of the working hand on the upper back just to the side of the spine and feel for the slight hollow where the fingertip fits naturally. Keep the finger straight, supporting it if necessary with the index finger and move the fingertip in small circles, moving the skin on the deeper tissue. Start quite lightly and gradually increase the depth. Work for five to ten circles before lifting the finger and moving down to the next hollow. The resting hand should be supporting the side of the back.

> ### REMEMBER
>
> *The fingers receive information, take note of any reaction such as tensing in the area being treated.*

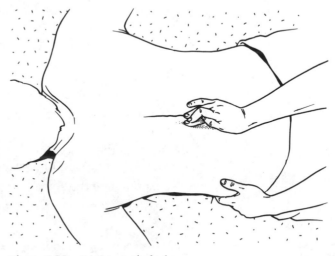

Figure 5.28   *Frictions to the back*

KEY TERMS

You need to know what these words mean. Go back through the chapter or look in the glossary to find out.

Distal	Prone	Supine
Effleurage	Stroking	Ulnar
Petrissage	Tapotement	

6 *The massage routine*

After working through this chapter you will be able to:

➤ prepare a client for a full body massage
➤ perform a full body massage using a suitable range of massage strokes
➤ determine and adapt the timing of massage for a whole body massage
➤ determine and adapt the timing of massage to particular areas
➤ obtain and appreciate the importance of client feedback.

In order to perform a body massage, the movements described in the previous chapter must be applied in some sort of order to the parts of the body to be treated. When starting to massage whole areas of the body rather than just practising a variety of strokes it is important to have a few basic rules to follow. In the main, the first type of massage to be mastered should be a classic general purpose massage as this is the type of massage which contains most of the strokes needed. Once you are proficient at this then it can be adapted for any other purpose.

For example a relaxing body massage is one where the majority of strokes are of the effleurage and stroking type with some petrissage, while a more stimulating massage will contain percussion movements and more vigorous petrissage. The speed and depth of the strokes will also vary from slow and relaxing to faster and more invigorating, but whatever the purpose of the massage the strokes must always show continuity and rhythm, and be at a depth suitable for the client being treated. The actual massage routine – that is the order of treating the parts of the body and the strokes used – is something that is altered to suit particular clients and to suit the preference of the therapist. Each expert massage therapist will have developed their own routines which are adapted and altered as part of a continual learning process. If you were to ask an expert to show you the massage movements that they used when they started, most would have difficulty in recalling them. However they would have initially have learnt the strokes, or very similar ones, described in the previous chapter and will have developed, varied, adapted and linked them together to make up massage routines for any part of the body.

The massage routine described in this chapter is a general 'all purpose' one which is suitable to learn initially, remembering that it can be altered and adapted to suit yourself and your client. It is a routine that uses the majority of the previously described strokes and therefore would have to be adapted to be a completely relaxing massage by leaving out the percussion movements and reducing the more vigorous petrissage movements.

Before attempting a full body massage the therapist should practise all the strokes on one particular part of the body until proficient before passing on to the next part. When you are proficient on each individual area then you can put it all together to perform a full body massage.

Whatever massage routine you will be performing, once it has started, that is once you have placed your hands on the clients body, then nothing should be allowed to disturb the continuity of the massage. This means of course that you must arrange your work so that you will not be disturbed by outside matters and that you have everything to hand so that you do not have to interrupt the massage to fetch anything. The preparation of the working area and the selection of suitable materials is described earlier, as is the consultation procedure. When everything is ready and the client is lying comfortably on the couch, then the massage can be started, remembering that only the part to be worked on should be uncovered as the rest of the body can quickly become chilled. Of course in very hot and humid climates this would not apply and here a very light cover can be used.

Timing a massage treatment can be very difficult and it takes a long time for it to become automatic. To begin with it is quite useful to time each individual part of the massage. If we assume that a full body massage will take an hour, not including the time taken for the client to prepare or to recover, then we can also suggest the time for each part within a routine. These times too of course will be altered and adapted to suit individual clients.

The following suggested routine is suitable to use to start with and can be adapted and altered to suit the client or your preference.

SUGGESTED OUTLINE and approximate times for a one hour massage

Client lies supine with head supported by a pillow.

1	Right leg	7 minutes
2	Left leg	7 minutes
3	Left arm	5 minutes
4	Chest	5 minutes
5	Right arm	5 minutes
6	Abdomen	5 minutes

Client turns over to lie prone, the pillow is removed.

7	Back of right leg including the buttock	5 minutes
8	Back of left leg including the buttock	5 minutes
9	Back and shoulders	15 minutes

This order of massage presumes that you are free to move around the couch as you wish. Occasionally, however, you might find yourself trying to carry out massage with a couch pushed up against a wall and then everything has to change!

Movement by the therapist should be kept to a minimum and wherever possible contact with the client maintained. In general the order of strokes to each area should be effleurage and stroking movements to

82

start, followed by a variety of petrissage movements, then percussion to suitable parts and effleurage and stroking to complete before moving on to the next section of the massage.

To start the general massage the client should be lying on the couch with support under the head and covered by towels in such a way as to allow access to each area of the body to be treated with as little disturbance as possible, one method is to have one towel lengthways across the top of the body and another lengthways along the legs and lower trunk.

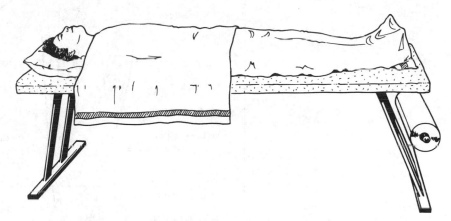

Figure 6.1 *Preparing the client for massage*

Numbers of repetitions of the strokes are not always given as this depends on the preference of the therapist and the specific needs of the client. To begin with you can aim to repeat each movement three or four times, so long as this fits into the timing for the area.

Leg massage

SUGGESTED MASSAGE MOVEMENTS for the right and left leg are:

1 Effleurage to the sides and front of the whole of the leg.
2 Effleurage to the thigh.
3 Double-handed kneading to the thigh.
4 Single-handed kneading to the thigh.
5 Wringing to the thigh muscles.
6 Hacking to the thigh muscles.
7 Stroking around the knee.
8 Effleurage to the back of the calf with knee bent.
9 Effleurage to the lower leg.
10 Thumb kneading to the anterior tibial muscles.
11 Effleurage to the foot.
12 Kneading to the sole of the foot.
13 Single-handed hacking to the sole of the foot.
14 Thumb stroking to top of foot.

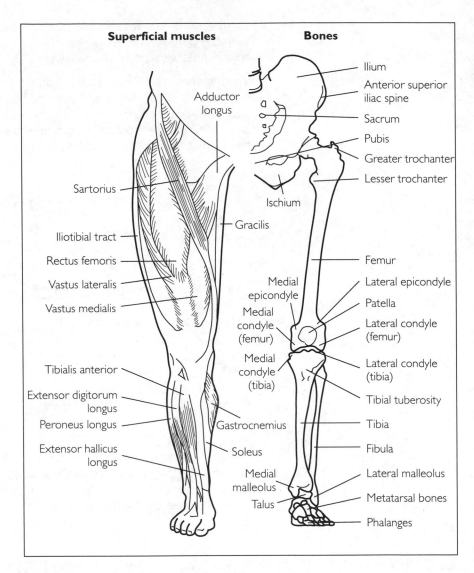

Superficial muscles

Adductor longus

Sartorius

Iliotibial tract

Rectus femoris

Vastus lateralis

Vastus medialis

Tibialis anterior

Extensor digitorum longus

Peroneus longus

Extensor hallicus longus

Gracilis

Medial epicondyle

Medial condyle (femur)

Medial condyle (tibia)

Gastrocnemius

Soleus

Medial malleolus

Talus

Bones

Ilium

Anterior superior iliac spine

Sacrum

Pubis

Greater trochanter

Lesser trochanter

Ischium

Femur

Lateral epicondyle

Patella

Lateral condyle (femur)

Lateral condyle (tibia)

Tibial tuberosity

Tibia

Fibula

Lateral malleolus

Metatarsal bones

Phalanges

Figure 6.2   *Muscles and bones of the front of the leg*

15 Thumb stroking across the sole of the foot.

16 Kneading to the toes.

17 Repeat of effleurage to the front and sides of the whole leg.

ACTIVITY	Before starting the massage remind yourself of the bony points to be avoided in the leg.

— REMEMBER —

Apply only enough oil to allow your hands to slide smoothly.

Fold the lower towel back to expose the whole of the right leg. Place some of the lubricant on the hands and apply it to the whole leg with sweeping, effleurage-type strokes.

1 Effleurage to the sides and front of leg

Stance   Walk-standing at the approximate level of the ankle making sure that you can reach to the top of the leg without straining.

Hands   Place the hands on the foot, one hand under the sole and the other on the top so that the foot is held between the hands.

Slide the hands firmly up the foot so that the top hand comes to the outside and the lower hand to the inside of the ankle and continue with the effleurage stroke up the inside and outside of the leg to the top of the thigh, when the outside hand sweeps firmly over the top of the leg towards the groin and the inguinal lymph nodes. Return the hands to the starting position by reversing the stroke but with much less pressure. Repeat two or three times.

The next effleurage stroke starts in the same way with the hands cradling the foot and then sliding up the sides of the lower leg, but just above the level of the knee they are brought in to overlap each other on top of the thigh and sweep up to the groin area. Return the hands to the starting position with one on the inside and the other on the outside of the leg in the same way and repeat two or three times.

— REMEMBER —

Move your weight from back foot to front foot to reach the top of the leg.

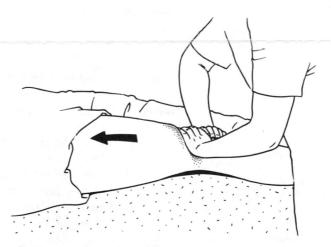

Figure 6.3   *Effleurage to the sides and front of leg*

2 Effleurage to the thigh

Stance   Walk-standing at a little below knee level.

a Hands   One inside and the other outside the thigh above the knee.

Effleurage as before from knee to groin with outer hand sweeping over the top of the thigh towards the inguinal nodes.

85

b Hands   Overlapping each other above the knee, sweeping up to groin and returning to the knee level on the inside and outside of the thigh.

3 Double-handed kneading to the thigh

(This movement is described on p. 62, Chapter 5.)

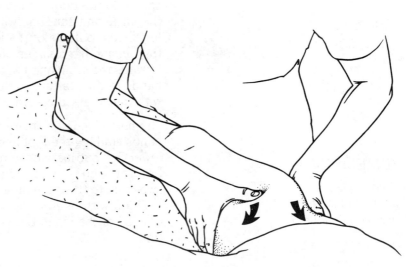

Figure 6.4   *Double-handed kneading to the thigh*

Stance   Walk-standing just below level of the knee.

Hands   Place one hand on the inside of the upper thigh and the other on the outside with the elbows bent and well away from the sides so that the thigh is squeezed between them. Move the hands alternately in circles away from you maintaining the squeezing effect and only moving over the skin to progress down the thigh to the knee. The hands can then slide back up the thigh to start again. Repeat two or three times.

4 Single-handed kneading to the thigh

(This movement is described on p. 61, Chapter 5.)

Stance   Walk-standing just below the level of the knee.

Hands   The working hand on the outside of the upper thigh and the other hand on the inner thigh for support.

The working hand is moved in a circular fashion on the outer thigh, moving the skin over the deeper tissues. The circle should be made three or four times before sliding

---

REMEMBER

Keep the whole hand in contact, but do not press too hard over the trochanter of the femur.

86

down a little to repeat the circling. When the level of the knee is reached the hand slides up to the start. Repeat two or three times.

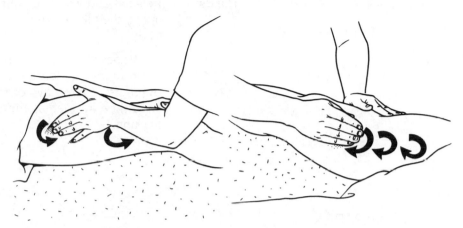

Figure 6.5   *Single-handed kneading to the thigh*

5 *Wringing to the muscles of the thigh*
(This movement is described on p. 66, Chapter 5.)

Stance   Walk or stride-standing facing across the client.

Hands   Placed on inner thigh facing each other with fingers together and thumbs apart.

Pick up the muscle on the inside of the thigh with one hand and then with the other and start the wringing movement by pulling with the fingers of one hand and pushing with the thumb of the other. The tissue is kept lifted from the bone as the hands wring and move up and down the thigh, first on the inside then on the top and then on the outside to cover the whole thigh.

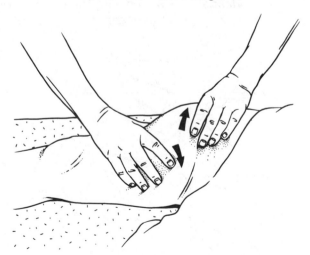

> — REMEMBER —
>
> *Bend your knees in order to reduce your height to work on the outside of the leg.*

Figure 6.6   *Wringing to the muscles of the thigh*

6 Hacking to the thigh muscles

Stance   Stride-standing facing across the client

Hands   Relaxed and with the palms facing each other a little way apart, the elbows should be bent and well away from the body.

Start hacking lightly down the front of the thigh and up again repeating so that the front and outer surface of the thigh are covered two or three times. The inner surface should be avoided as the tissue can be too sensitive for hacking.

REMEMBER

Only the backs of the little, ring and middle fingers are used with a small part of the ulnar border of the hand.
The movement should be a quick, light, flicking one.

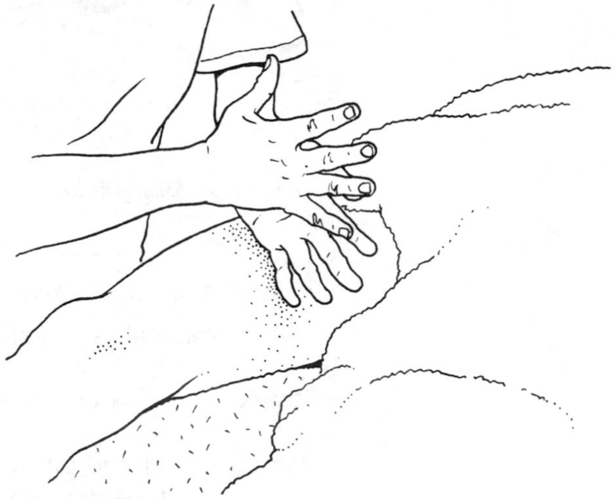

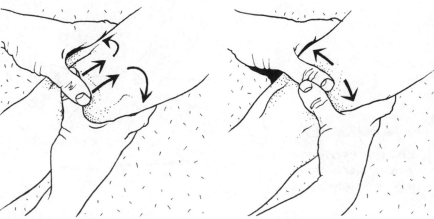

Figure 6.7   *Hacking to the thigh muscles*

Before moving on to the knee, effleurage over the thigh once or twice.

7 Stroking around the knee

Stance   Walk-standing below knee level.

Hands   Placed with the thumbs overlapping below the patella and the fingers resting at the sides of the knee.

Figure 6.8   *Stroking around the knees*

The thumbs stroke lightly up over the patella and then sweep firmly around the edges of the patella and down towards the back of the knee to meet the fingers at the sides. Repeat two or three times.

8 Effleurage to the back of the calf

With one hand under the heel and the other supporting the knee, bend the leg up to a 90 degree angle and rest the heel on the bed.

Stance   Walk-standing at ankle level

Hands   One above the other on the back of the leg at ankle level with the elbows well away from the sides of the body.

One hand is moved firmly up the calf and as it reaches to just below the knee, the other hand moves in the same way so that one hand is always moving and the other returning to the starting position. This can be repeated five or six times.

Return the leg to the lying position by supporting it at the knee and the heel.

<table>
<tr><td>— REMEMBER —

Always support joints such as the knee when moving a limb.</td></tr>
</table>

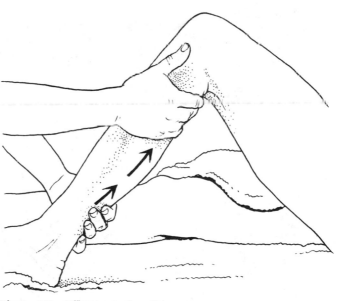

Figure 6.9   *Effleurage to the calf*

9 Effleurage to the lower leg

Stance   Walk-standing at level of the foot.

Hands   Cradling the foot as in the first effleurage movement.

Effleurage up the sides of the lower leg as far as the knee and return with a lighter stroking movement. Repeat two or three times.

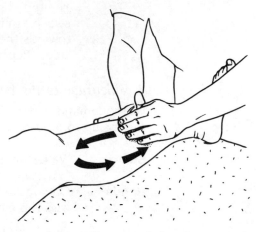

Figure 6.10   *Effleurage to the lower leg*

10 *Thumb kneading to the anterior tibial muscles*

Stance   Walk-standing at ankle level.

Hands   The working hand is placed on the outer side of the lower leg, just below the knee, with the other hand acting as a support on the inner surface.

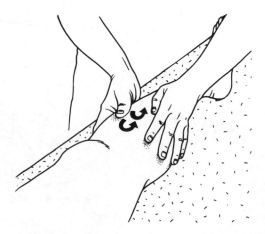

Figure 6.11   *Thumb kneading to the anterior tibial muscle*

REMEMBER

Avoid the anterior surface of the tibia which is just under the skin.

The working hand kneads with the thumb in small circles down the outer surface to just above the ankle. Then the hand returns with an effleurage stroke to the beginning. Repeat once or twice.

11 Effleurage to the foot

Stance   Walk-standing below foot level.

Hands   One on the upper surface to support and the other, the working hand, on the sole, both facing the same way.

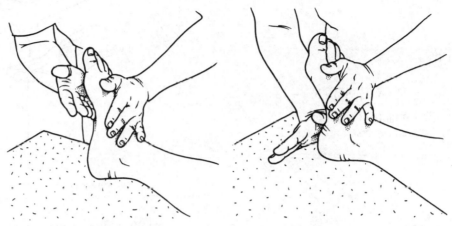

Figure 6.12 *Effleurage to the foot*   **Figure 6.13** *Effleurage to the foot*

With the working hand fitting close into the sole of the foot, effleurage deeply from base of toes to the heel.

12 Kneading to the sole of the foot

Stance   Walk-standing below foot level.

Hands   One on the upper surface to support and the other, the working hand, on the sole, both facing the same way.

Using the base of the thumb area to create pressure, perform circular kneading movements up and down the sole of the foot.

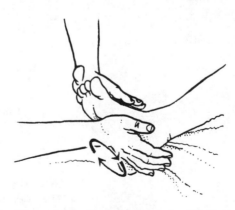

Figure 6.14 *Kneading to the sole of the foot*

91

13 *Single-handed hacking to the sole of the foot*

Stance   Walk-standing below foot level.

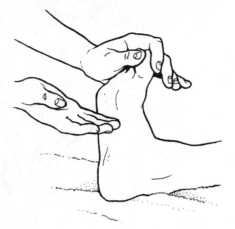

Figure 6.15   *Single-handed hacking to the sole of the foot*

─── REMEMBER ───
Use only the sides of the
relaxed fingers.

Hands   With one hand supporting the upper surface of the foot, use the other hand to lightly hack over the arched part of the sole.

14 *Thumb stroking to the top of the foot*

Stance   Walk-standing below foot level.

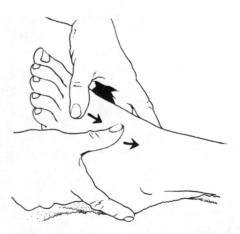

Figure 6.16   *Thumb stroking to the top of the foot*

Hands   Fingers under the foot and the thumbs on top.

With the thumbs, stroke the top of the foot from the base of the toes upwards. The thumbs should stroke along the spaces between all the long metatarsal bones of the foot .

92

REMEMBER

When handling the foot firmness is important to avoid tickling.

15 *Thumb stroking across the sole of the foot*

Stance   Walk-standing below foot level.

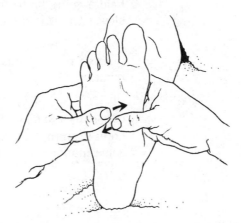

Figure 6.17   *Thumb stroking across the sole of the foot*

Hands   Fingers on top of the foot and the thumbs under the foot lying across the sole.

Move the arms so that the thumbs move firmly across the sole of the foot, crossing and uncrossing. Repeat the movement as the hands slide down from toes to heel.

16 *Kneading to the toes*

Stance   Walk-standing below foot level.

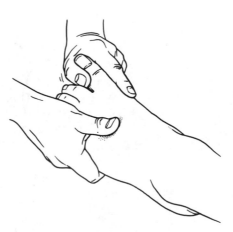

Figure 6.18   *Kneading to the toes*

Hands   Each toe in turn is grasped.

Each toe is gently grasped and rolled between the thumb and forefinger and at the same time gently pulled.

17 Effleurage to the whole leg

Complete the leg massage by repeating the first effleurage strokes to the whole leg, to the front and to the sides. As these are the last movements before going on to the next part of the body they should get lighter and slower towards the end.

PROGRESS CHECK   Practise the leg massage until you can perform it fluently within 7–8 minutes.

Cover the right leg. Walk around the base of the couch to remove the cover from the left leg and proceed to massage the left leg in exactly the same manner. Then proceed to the arm massage.

Arm massage (left)

Although the pattern of movements on the arm are similar to those on the leg, the technique needs to be different. The leg is a heavy limb which will stay in place as you carry out the manipulations, whereas the arm is much lighter. Neither is the arm so densely covered in muscle.

There are a number of ways in which the arm can be supported during massage and as a therapist you will find your own preferred method. The arm may be supported by one of your hands and rest along one arm while the other hand works, or the arm may lie on the bed while you use both hands to work. A mixture of these two methods will be described.

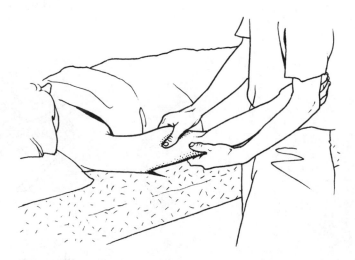

Figure 6.19 *Supporting the arm*

In general the pattern of movements is similar in that effleurage movements start and finish the massage with petrissage and percussion in between.

94

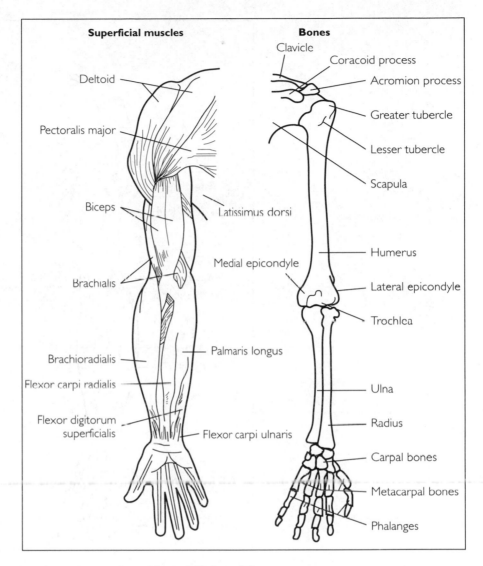

Figure 6.20 *Muscles and bones of the front of the arm*

SUGGESTED MASSAGE MOVEMENTS for the arm are:

1 Effleurage to the posterior aspect of the arm.
2 Effleurage to the anterior aspect of the arm.
3 Single-handed picking up to the deltoid and triceps muscles.
4 Single-handed picking up to the biceps muscle.
5 Wringing to the whole upper arm.
6 Light hacking to the upper arm.
7 Effleurage to the forearm.
8 Single-handed picking up to the forearm muscles.
9 Thumb stroking to the palm of the hand.
10 Thumb kneading to thenar (thumb) muscles and the hypothenar (little finger) muscles.

95

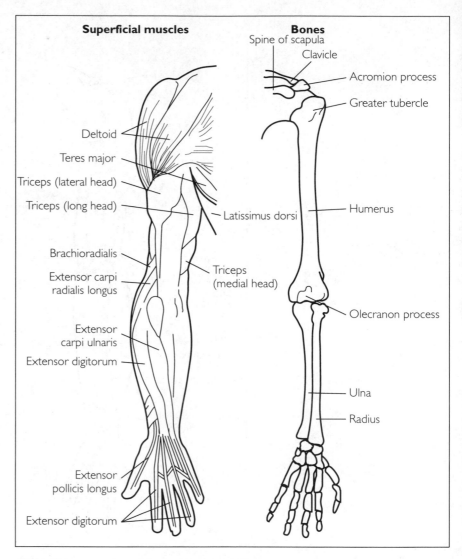

Figure 6.21 *Muscles and bones of the back of the arm*

11 Kneading to individual fingers and thumb with stretching.
12 Thumb stroking to back of hand.
13 Circular thumb kneading to the back of the hand.
14 Repeat the effleurage to the front and back of the whole arm.

To start, fold back the towel to expose the arm.

1 *Effleurage to the posterior aspect of the arm*

Stance   Walk-standing in direction of stroke.

Hands   The left hand supports the upper arm near the axilla (armpit) so that the whole arm and hand of the client lies on the left arm of the therapist. This leaves the right hand free to work.

With the right hand moulded over the hand, effleurage up to and around the shoulder, returning to the hand with a lighter stroke. Repeat two or three times.

2 Effleurage to the anterior aspect of the arm

Stance   Walk-standing in direction of stroke.

Hands   The arm is turned to rest on the right hand and arm of the therapist whose left hand is now free to work. With the left hand moulded to the part, effleurage firmly up to the axilla and lightly down.

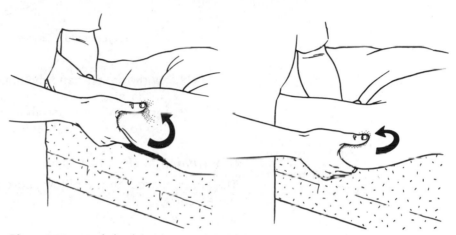

Figure 6.22   *Single-handed picking up of the deltoid and triceps muscles*

3 Single-handed picking up to the deltoid and triceps muscles

Stance   Walk-standing in direction of stroke.

Hands   As in movement 1, Effleurage to the posterior aspect of the arm, so that the right hand is free to work and the client's arm is supported.

With the right hand moulded over the upper part of the deltoid muscle at the top of the arm, pick up the muscle from the bone, squeeze, release and move down a little. When the hand reaches the lower part of deltoid, slide it back a little to cover the triceps muscle and pick up until the hand reaches a level of just above the elbow. Slide the hand up to reach the top of the arm and repeat a number of times.

4 Single-handed picking up of biceps

Stance   Walk-standing in direction of stroke.

Hands   As in movement 2, Effleurage to the anterior aspect of the arm, so that the client's arm is supported and your left hand is free to work.

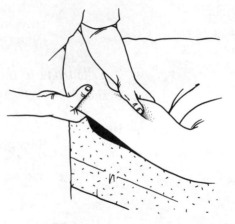

Figure 6.23 *Single-handed picking up of the biceps*

With the left hand moulded over the biceps just below the axilla pick up, squeeze and release, moving the hand down gradually until just above the elbow. Slide the hand firmly up to the top and repeat.

5 *Wringing to the upper arm*

The arm is placed on the pillow above the client's head for this movement.

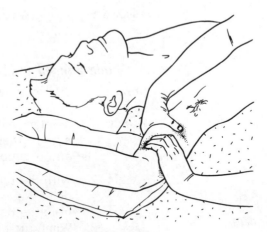

Figure 6.24 *Wringing to the upper arm*

Stance	Stride-standing to face across the client.
Hands	Both working, facing each other, with elbows well out to the side.
	Alternate hands lift the tissue, squeeze it and the fingers of one hand pull it towards you while the thumb of the other hand pushes it away. The hands wring up and down the upper arm to cover all the accessible muscle tissue.

6 Light hacking over the upper arm

The arm can be placed by the side of the body.

Stance   Stride-standing to face across the client.

Hands   Both working, with palms facing each other and elbows well out.

Lightly hack over the accessible muscle tissue using the outer surface of the little, ring and middle fingers only, not the border of the hand.

> ### REMEMBER
>
> *The depth of the hacking depends on the density of the tissue.*

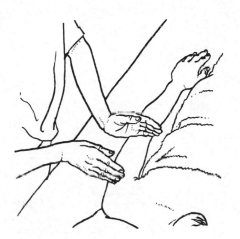

Figure 6.25   *Light hacking over the upper arm*

7 Effleurage to the forearm

Stance   Walk-standing facing the head of the couch.

Hands   The left hand holds the hand of the client so that the client's elbow is bent and resting on the bed.

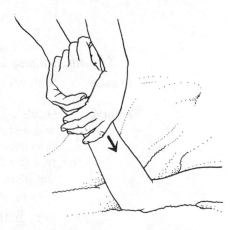

Figure 6.26   *Effleurage to the forearm*

With the right hand moulded around the forearm at wrist level, effleurage firmly down to the elbow, then stroke lightly up to repeat two or three times.

8 Single-handed picking up to the forearm

Stance   Walk-standing facing the head of the couch.

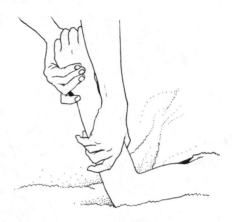

Figure 6.27   Single-handed picking up to the forearm

Hands   The left hand holds the hand of the client so that the client's elbow is bent and resting on the bed.

With the right hand moulded around the forearm at wrist level, pick up and release the tissue at the side of the forearm. Work towards the elbow, then back to the wrist, picking up the muscles on the front of the forearm.

9 Thumb stroking to the palm

Stance   Walk-standing facing across the client.

Hands   Holding the client's hand so that the elbow is slightly bent and resting on the bed. The therapist places one little finger between the thumb and forefinger of the client's hand so that the thumb is held out of the way and the other between the little finger and ring finger. The therapist's thumbs can now lie on the palm of the hand.

With both thumbs, stroke the palms firmly from base of fingers to the wrist.

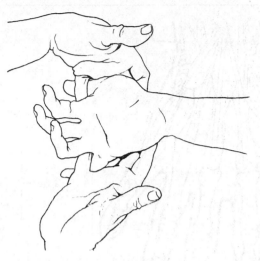

Figure 6.28 *Supporting the hand for thumb stroking and kneading to the palm*

10 Thumb kneading to the thenar and hypothenar muscles

Stance   Walk-standing facing across the client.

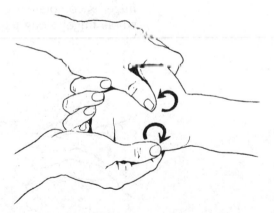

Figure 6.29 *Thumb kneading to the thenar and hypothenar muscles*

Hands   As for movement 9, Thumb stroking to the palm.

Both thumbs perform circular kneading movements over the muscular tissue.

11 Kneading to individual fingers

Stance   Walk-standing facing across the client.

Hands   One hand supports the client's hand at the wrist.

101

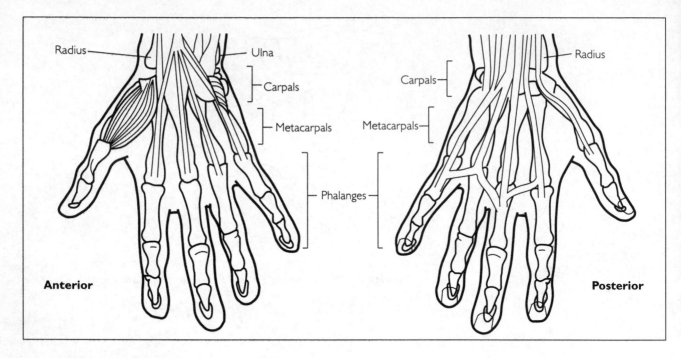

Figure 6.30 *Structure of the hand*

Each finger is taken in turn and kneaded from base to tip between the fingers and thumb of the therapist. As each finger is completed, gentle traction is applied, holding the whole finger along its length.

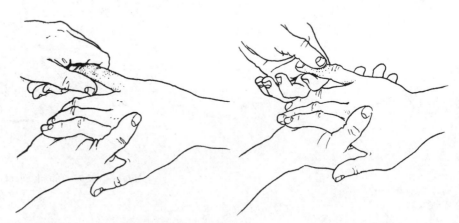

Figure 6.31 *Kneading to individual fingers*

12 *Thumb stroking to the back of the hand*

Stance   Walk-standing facing across the client.

Hands   Both supporting the client's hand with the back of the hand facing upwards.

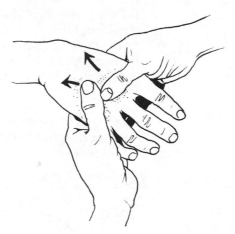

Figure 6.32 *Thumb stroking to the back of the hand*

With the tips of the thumbs running between the metacarpal bones, stroke firmly up towards the wrist.

13 *Circular thumb kneading to the back of the hand*

Stance   Walk-standing facing across the client

Hands   As for movement 12, Thumb stroking to the back of the hand.

Taking care not to press too hard on the metacarpals, perform small, circular kneading movements up and down the back of the hand with both thumbs.

14 *Effleurage to front and back of the whole arm*

Repeat the effleurage movements to the whole arm as described in movements 1 and 2.

The arm should be placed under the towel before continuing the massage.

PROGRESS CHECK	Practise the arm massage until it is fluent and can be performed within 5–6 minutes.

Chest massage

The preferred position for the therapist during this short part of the body massage is at the head of the bed. If this is not possible then movements may be adapted to be performed from one side.

The towel covering the upper part of the body should be folded back to expose the upper chest and shoulders. This is also a good opportunity to remove any pillows from under the client's head, allowing greater access to the neck and shoulder region.

Care must be taken during massage to this area as the tissue is generally sensitive. Effleurage and suitable petrissage movements are used but rarely any percussion. Although this is a chest massage, the position of the body allows quite deep massage to the back of the neck and shoulders and these should be integrated into this part of the treatment.

ACTIVITY	Remind yourself of the arrangement of the bones and muscles of the chest and upper back.

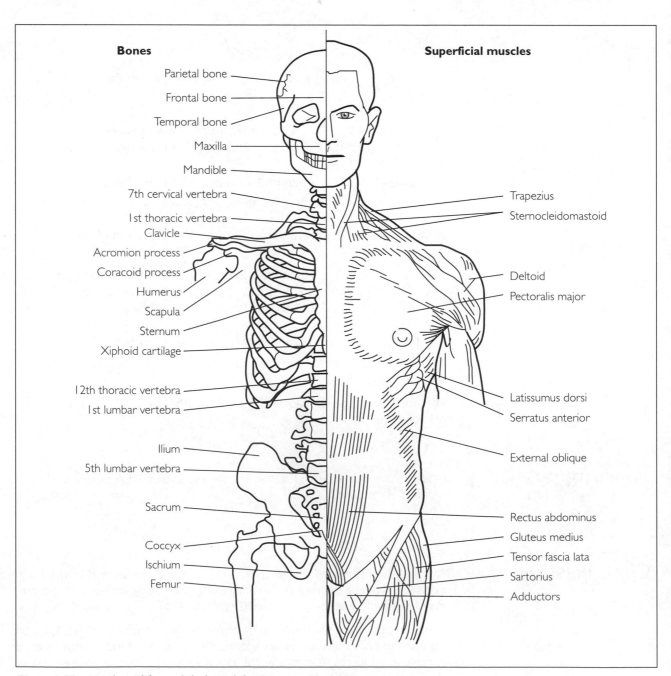

Figure 6.33 *Muscles and bones of the front of the torso*

Use the first effleurage strokes to apply the massage medium to the whole area.

SUGGESTED MASSAGE MOVEMENTS for the chest are:

1 Effleurage to chest and back of neck with slight traction.
2 Stroking to one side of the neck with alternate hands.
3 Stroking to the other side of the neck with alternate hands.
4 Finger kneading to the upper fibres of the trapezius muscle from shoulders to the base of the skull.

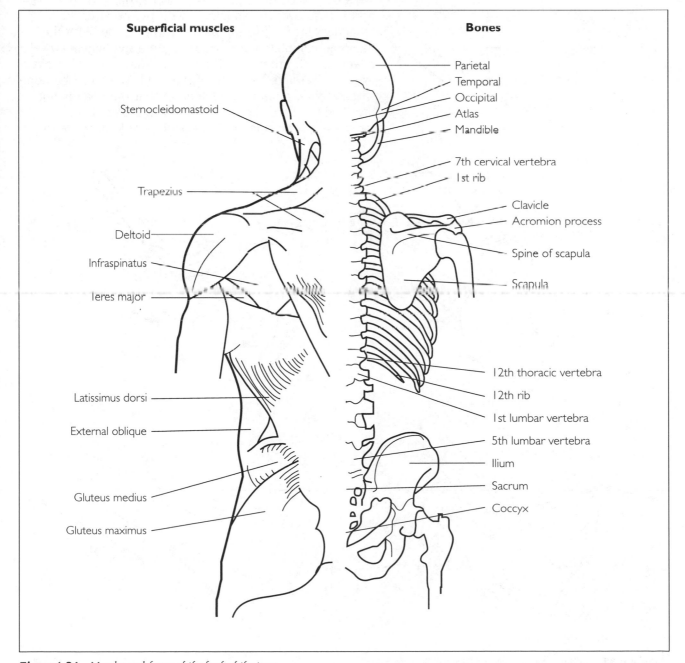

Figure 6.34   *Muscles and bones of the back of the torso*

5 Kneading to the front of the chest and shoulders.

6 Effleurage to chest and back of neck.

1 *Effleurage to the chest and back of neck with slight traction*

Stance Walk-standing at the head of the couch.

Hands Both hands are placed side by side on the sternum.

Stroke down the chest just far enough not to impinge on breast tissue, then, turning your hands to point outwards, glide the hands over the chest towards the shoulders. The hands pass over the shoulders with the point of the shoulders fitting into the palms of the hands. With the hands in complete contact all the time the fingers swivel towards each other onto the back of the neck and stroke firmly upwards to the base of the skull. This must be done with a gentle pulling movement so that the head is not lifted off the bed. The hands return to the start with a light stroke down the side of the neck. Repeat four or five times.

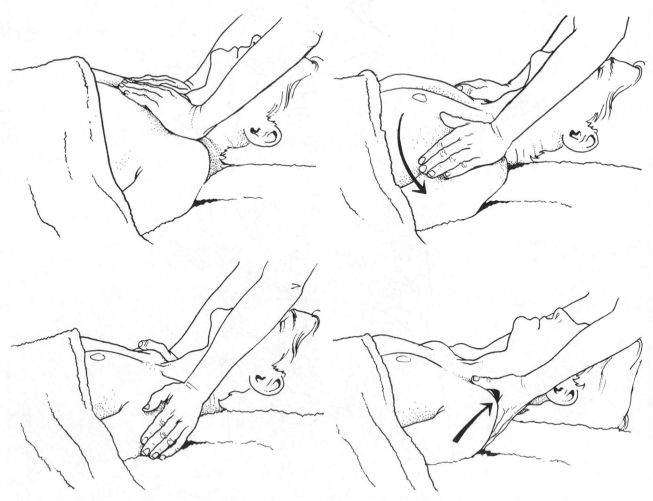

Figure 6.35 *Effleurage to the chest and back of the neck*

2 Stroking to one side of the neck with alternate hands

Stance   Walk-standing at the head of the couch.

Hands   One hand cupped over the shoulder near the point of the shoulder.

Stroke firmly up the side of the neck to the base of the skull behind the ear, as it reaches the skull follow it with the other hand in exactly the same way,. One of the hands should always be in contact as the other is returning to the start. The hands should be pointing down towards the bed during this movement and should be kept away from the front of the neck. Repeat several times.

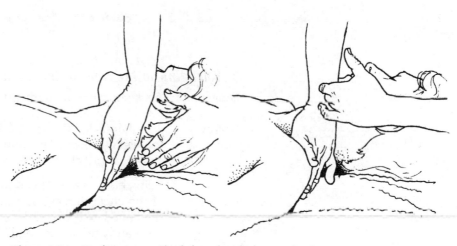

Figure 6.36   *Stroking to one side of the neck with alternate hands*

3 Repeat stroking to the other side of the neck

Repeat the strokes of massage movement 2 on the other side of the neck.

4 Finger kneading to the upper fibres of trapezius

Stance   Walk-standing at the head of the couch.

Hands   Under the shoulders, palm up, with the fingertips on the muscle.

With both hands working, use the fingertips for firm, circular kneading movements along the muscle towards the centre, then up the back of the neck at the sides of the spine to the base of the skull. Slide the hands down to the start and repeat twice.

— REMEMBER —

Don't work over the bony points of the shoulder.

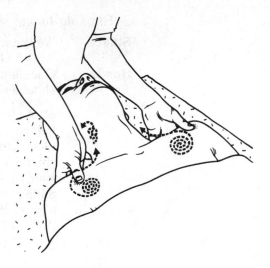

Figure 6.37 *Finger kneading to upper fibres of trapezius*

5 Kneading to the front of the chest and shoulders

Stance   Walk-standing at the head of the couch.

Hands   With hands lightly clenched, place the flat part of the fingers (between the knuckles and fingertips) of both hands on the centre of the chest side by side.

Using both hands, knead in circles very gently over the front of the chest moving outwards towards the shoulders. Move the hands, still kneading, over the deltoid muscle then open the hands to sweep behind the shoulders and neck. Return to the start and repeat.

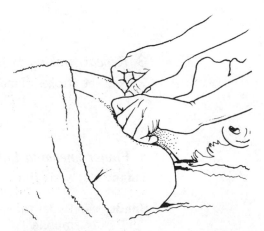

Figure 6.38 *Kneading to the front of the chest and shoulders*

6 Effleurage to the chest and back of the neck

Repeat the effleurage strokes of movement 1, but with less traction.

PROGRESS CHECK Practise until the chest massage can be completed fluently in 5 minutes.

Unfold the towel so that it covers the chest area and exposes the right arm.

Arm massage (right)

The massage strokes are a repeat of those used on the left arm, though the therapist's working hand changes. For example, where the right hand previously supported the left arm while the left hand worked, now the left hand does the supporting while the right hand works.

Finish the arm by covering it with the towel and expose the abdomen by folding back the upper and lower towels.

Abdomen massage

SAFE PRACTICE ▷ *The abdomen should only be included in the body massage if the therapist is sure that it is appropriate. The specific contra-indication is pregnancy, especially during the early months. In the last months of pregnancy some gentle effleurage movements may be performed over the abdominal wall, but only after consultation with the client's medical advisors.*

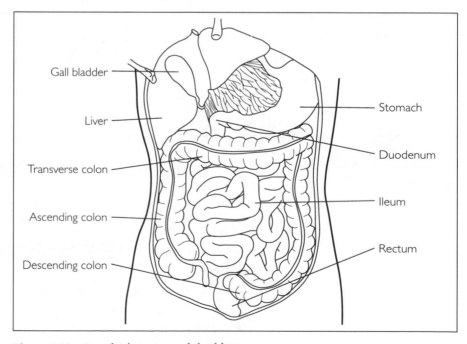

Figure 6.39 *Superficial structures of the abdomen*

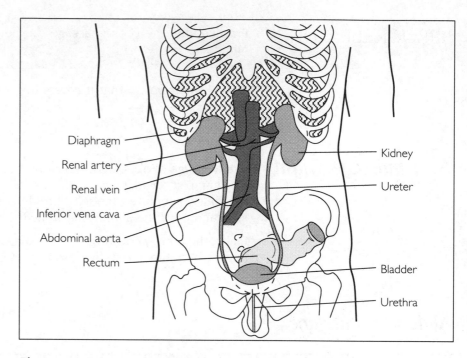

Figure 6.40 *Deep structures of the abdomen*

Many female clients prefer not to have the abdomen worked over during their menstrual period and this should always be respected. Others look to a massage to relieve the discomfort felt in the first days of menstruation and so long as the movements are gentle and the client warned that the menstrual flow may be increased, there should be no problem.

It is often helpful to place a rolled up towel under the client's knees so that the abdominal wall is relaxed.

GOOD PRACTICE ▷ *Therapists should avoid working on the abdominal area of a client of the opposite sex.*

SUGGESTED MASSAGE MOVEMENTS for the abdomen are:

1 Effleurage to the abdomen.
2 Circular stroking to the abdomen.
3 Circular kneading over the colon.
4 Wringing to the sides and front of the abdomen.
5 Effleurage to the abdomen.

110

1 *Effleurage to the abdomen*

Stance Walk-standing close to the couch at the level of the client's hip.

Hands Placed side by side on the front of the abdomen above the pubis. Without applying much pressure, move the hands upwards until the fingers reach the bottom of the sternum, then turn the hands to point down towards the bed and continue to sweep down over the ribs, down the side of the waist, and then bring them up inside the iliac crest, wrists first, to the starting point. This is a very relaxing stroke and can be repeated four or five times, increasing the pressure slightly.

┌─ REMEMBER ─┐
Don't press down into the
abdomen.

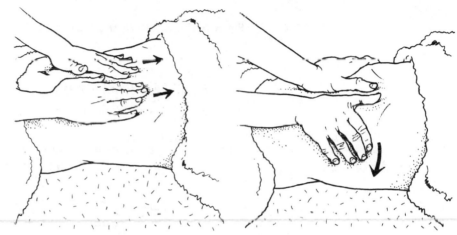

Figure 6.41 *Effleurage to the abdomen*

2 *Circular stroking to the abdomen*

Stance Walk-standing close to the couch at the level of the client's hip.

┌─ REMEMBER ─┐
Keep the pressure even.

Hands The main working hand is placed flat on the abdomen to one side just below the ribs with the other placed slightly behind it.

The first hand strokes in a large circle over the colon in a clockwise direction, up the right side, across the top and down the left side of the abdomen. This hand stays in contact all the time while circling. The other hand follows the main working hand but has to cross over the working hand to complete the circle.

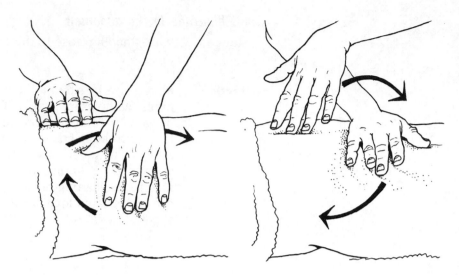

Figure 6.42 *Circular stroking to the abdomen*

3 Circular kneading over the colon

Stance   Walk-standing close to the couch at the level of the client's hip.

Hands   Main working hand in same starting position as for movement 2, Circular stroking to the abdomen, but with the other hand placed lightly on top.

Following the same clockwise direction, small circular kneading movements are performed over the colon.

— REMEMBER —

Don't press over the bladder.

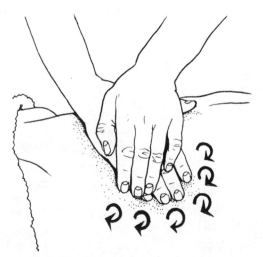

Figure 6.43 *Circular kneading over the colon*

4 Wringing to sides and front of abdomen

Stance   Walk-standing facing across the client.

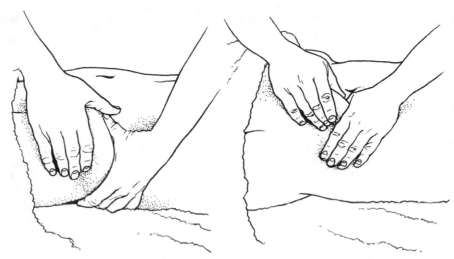

Figure 6.44 *Wringing to the sides and front of the abdomen*

Hands Placed facing each other on the far side of the waist Pick up the tissue on the far side of the waist and wring up and down the waist, front of abdomen and the near side of the waist, repeating three or four times.

5 Effleurage to the abdomen

Repeat the first effleurage stroke four or five times. As this is the end of the massage to the front of the body make the effleurage movements slower and slower and at the end, cup your hands over the navel. The warmth from your hands is a comforting end to this part of the massage.

PROGRESS CHECK Practise until you can perform the abdominal massage in 4–5 minutes.

Remove the rolled towel from under the knees and ask the client to turn over into the prone position, holding the towels in position. Any remaining pillows should be removed so that the head lies flat.

Back of right leg (including buttock)

The lower towel is folded back to expose the whole of the leg and buttock region. It is usually of benefit to place a small rolled up towel under the ankle of the leg to be worked on. This helps the muscles on the back of the leg to relax and stops the foot being pressed onto the bed which would be uncomfortable.

SUGGESTED MASSAGE MOVEMENTS for the back of the leg are:

1 Effleurage to the back of the leg and buttock.
2 Effleurage to the thigh and buttock.
3 Single-handed kneading to the outer surface of the thigh.

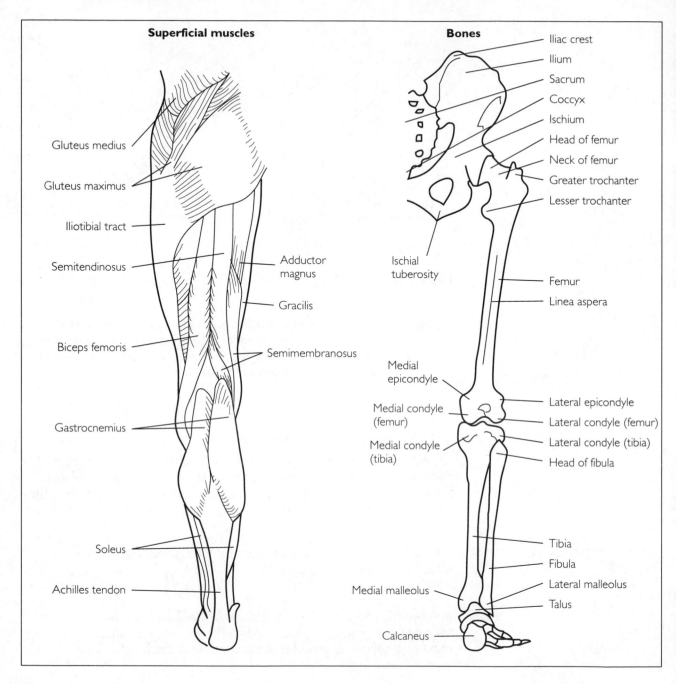

Superficial muscles

Gluteus medius

Gluteus maximus

Iliotibial tract

Semitendinosus

Biceps femoris

Gastrocnemius

Soleus

Achilles tendon

Adductor magnus

Gracilis

Semimembranosus

Bones

Iliac crest

Ilium

Sacrum

Coccyx

Ischium

Head of femur

Neck of femur

Greater trochanter

Lesser trochanter

Ischial tuberosity

Femur

Linea aspera

Medial epicondyle

Medial condyle (femur)

Medial condyle (tibia)

Lateral epicondyle

Lateral condyle (femur)

Lateral condyle (tibia)

Head of fibula

Tibia

Fibula

Lateral malleolus

Talus

Medial malleolus

Calcaneus

Figure 6.45 *Muscles and bones of the back of the leg*

4 Reinforced kneading to buttock and back of thigh.

5 Wringing over the buttock and back of thigh.

6 Double-handed picking up over the hamstring muscles.

7 Hacking over buttocks and back of thigh.

8 Beating over buttocks and back of thigh.

9 Clapping over buttocks and back of thigh.

10 Effleurage to buttock and thigh.

11 Effleurage to calf.

12 Wringing to calf muscles.

13 Light hacking to calf.

14 Effleurage to back of leg and buttock.

1 Effleurage to the back of the leg and buttock

Stance   Walk-standing at a level which allows the therapist to reach the whole length of the leg.

Hands   The inner hand should be on the sole of the foot and the outer hand on the outer surface of the ankle.

Both hands effleurage firmly up the leg, over the buttock with the hands sweeping to the outer surface of the hip towards the groin to finish the stroke before returning to the start. Repeat four or five times.

2 Effleurage to the thigh and buttock

Stance   Walk-standing at knee level.

Hands   Placed one above the other, above the knee across the thigh.

Sweep both hands up the thigh and over the buttocks where they separate and return to the start down the sides of the thigh.

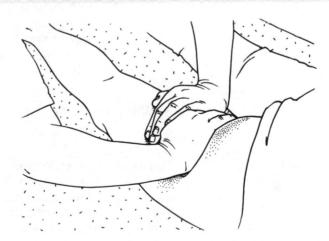

Figure 6.46   *Effleurage to the thigh and buttock*

REMEMBER

Don't press too hard over the greater trochanter of the femur.

3 Single-handed kneading to outer surface of the thigh

Stance   Walk-standing at knee level.

Hands   The outer, working hand is placed on the outer surface of the hip and the inner hand rests on and supports the thigh.

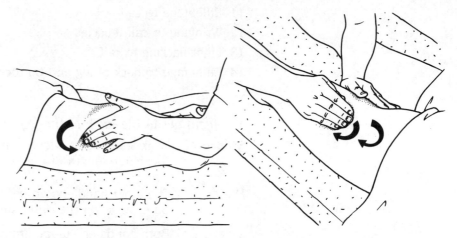

Figure 6.47 *Single-handed kneading to the outer surface of the thigh*

With the outer hand, knead in circles, moving gradually down the thigh to just above the knee. Then work in the same way up the thigh again.

4 Reinforced kneading to the buttock and back of thigh

Stance   Walk-standing at knee level

Hands   Working hand flat on the buttock with the other hand resting on it.

With circular movements, knead over the buttock area taking care not to pull the buttocks apart, then down the back of the thigh to just above the knee. Use a sweeping effleurage stroke to return to the start. Repeat once.

5 Wringing to the buttock and back of thigh

Stance   Walk or stride-standing facing across the client.

Hands   Placed on the inner thigh just above the knee with fingers together and thumbs apart. Wring in the same way as on the front of the leg, working up the thigh, over the buttock and down, until the whole thigh and buttock is covered. Repeat once or twice.

6 Double-handed picking up over the back of the thigh

Stance   Walk-standing facing up the body

Hands   Placed high on the thigh forming a wide V shape with the thumb of one hand alongside the index finger of the other hand.

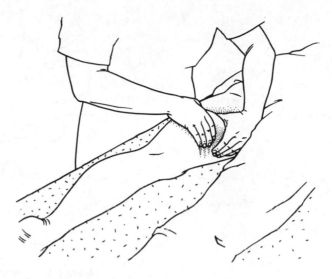

Figure 6.48   *Wringing to the back of leg and thigh*

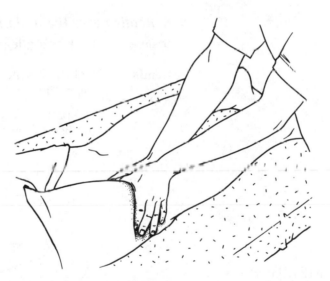

Figure 6.49   *Double-handed picking up over the back of the thigh*

Squeeze the muscles between both hands, lift and release and move the hands lower down. Repeat, moving up and down the thigh, covering the whole area two or three times.

7 Hacking to the buttocks and back of the thigh

Stance   Walk or stride-standing facing across body.

Hands   Relaxed and with the palms facing each other a little way apart and the elbows held well away from the sides.

Start hacking lightly down the back of the thigh and up again to cover the whole of the buttocks and back and outer surface of the thigh two or three times.

117

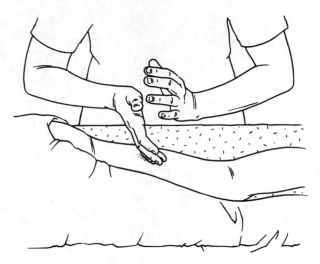

Figure 6.50 *Hacking to the buttocks and the back of the thigh*

8 Beating over the buttocks and back of the thigh

Stance   Walk or stride-standing facing across the body.

Hands   Lightly clenched, held side by side above the surface of the thigh. The wrists should be very loose.

Whats   The part is struck with alternate hands using the flat part of the fist. Cover the part two or three times.

REMEMBER

Most of the movement for beating takes place at the wrists.

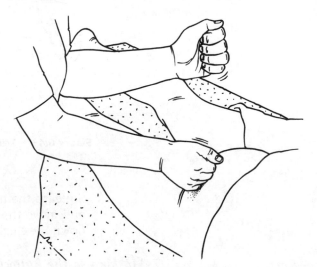

Figure 6.51 *Beating over the buttocks and the back of the thigh*

9 Clapping over the buttocks and back of the thigh

Stance   Walk or stride-standing facing across the body.

Hands   Cupped, with fingers straight and thumbs close in to the side of the fingers.

118

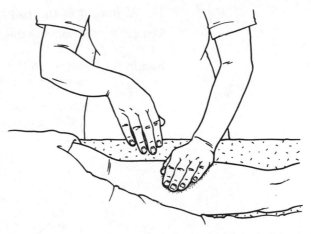

Figure 6.52 *Clapping over the buttocks and the back of the thigh*

The hands strike the part alternately, producing a dull, hollow sound, not a slap. The whole of the back of the thigh and buttock may be covered once or twice.

10 Effleurage over buttock and thigh

Repeat the strokes of movement 2.

11 Effleurage to the calf

Stance   Walk-standing at ankle level.

Hands   One above the other, lying across the calf above the ankle.

Both hands sweep upwards as far as the knee and separate for the return, downward strokes on the outer surfaces of the lower leg.

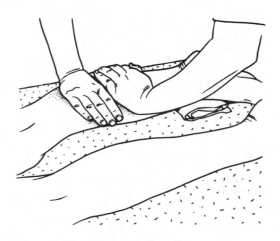

Figure 6.53 *Effleurage to the calf*

119

12 Wringing to the calf

Stance Stride-standing facing across the body.

Hands Placed on the calf, facing each other with the fingers together and thumbs apart.

Wring the calf muscles up and down between knee and ankle. Cover the whole area two or three times.

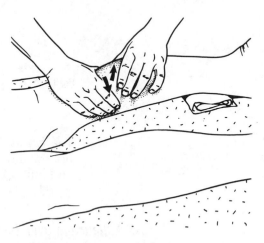

Figure 6.54 Wringing to the calf

13 Light hacking to the calf

Stance Stride-standing facing across the body.

Hands Relaxed with palms facing each other a little way apart and the elbows held well away from the sides.

Lightly hack up and down the calf, covering the whole area two or three times.

REMEMBER

If there is any evidence of varicose veins in the area, only the light effleurage should be used.

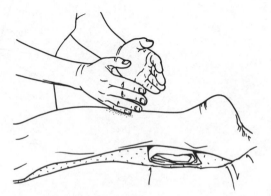

Figure 6.55 Light hacking to the calf

14 *Effleurage to the back of leg and buttocks*

Repeat the strokes of movement 1. As this is the last movement in this part of the massage, it should be performed so that the movements get slower and lighter towards the end.

When both legs are completed, cover the legs with towels, making sure that the feet are covered, and fold down the top towel to expose the back from the shoulders to the level of the top of the sacrum.

Back massage

Look at Figure 6.34 to remind yourself of the bones and muscles of the back.

Very occasionally a client may benefit from a small pillow or folded towel under the abdomen during this part of the massage. For instance, clients with a very hollow back or with large breasts will be able to lie prone with more comfort with support under the abdomen.

The client's hands may be placed under the forehead or at the sides. If they are under the forehead, the elbows should be quite low to allow the therapist to massage the shoulder area.

The back is the last part of the body to be massaged in this routine and as such is the part that will make the final impression on the client. The back is a large area with many bony points to be avoided or treated with care. The muscles of the back tend to become very tense and should benefit a great deal from the massage.

SUGGESTED MASSAGE MOVEMENTS for the back are:

1 Reverse effleurage.
2 T-shaped effleurage.
3 Circular stroking around left and right scapulae.
4 Figure of eight reinforced stroking around the scapulae.
5 Flat-handed kneading to the whole back.
6 Single-handed picking up to back of neck.
7 Wringing to shoulders and tops of arms.
8 Finger kneading/frictions at the sides of the spine.
9 T-shaped effleurage.
10 Effleurage towards lymph nodes (lower cervical, axillary and inguinal).
11 Wringing to sides of back.
12 Skin rolling to sides of back.
13 Transverse stroking to the lumbar region.
14 Light hacking over whole back.
15 T-shaped effleurage.

Before starting the back massage, remind yourself of the bony points and the arrangement of the muscles in the back.

1 Reverse effleurage

Stance   Walk or stride-standing at the head of the couch, standing close enough to the couch to be able to reach the whole length of the back.

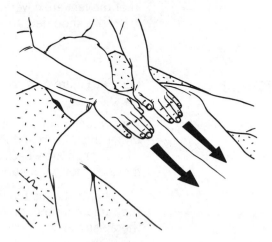

Figure 6.56   *Reverse effleurage*

Hands   Placed flat on the upper back, one on each side of the spine.

The hands are moved downwards to the base of the spine, then moved to the sides of the hips and glide firmly up the sides of the back to resume the starting position. The upward movement should be firmer than the downward one.

SAFE PRACTICE ▷ *Protect your back by not stretching further than you can easily reach. A short therapist may like to omit this movement.*

Keeping one hand in contact with the body for the sake of continuity, move around to the side of the couch.

2 T-shaped effleurage

Stance   Walk – standing at a level allowing you to reach the whole length of the back. Choose the side of the couch which is best for you. A right-handed therapist will usually choose to work from the left side of the client.

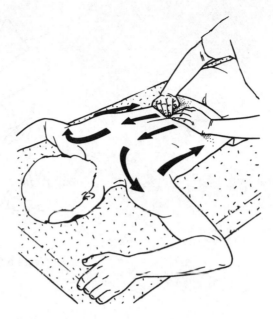

Figure 6.57 T-shaped effleurage

Hands   Flat on the back at the base of the spine, one hand on each side of the spine.

Effleurage firmly up the sides of the spine to the base of the neck, slide outwards to the shoulders, over the upper arms, back to the shoulders and down the sides of the back to the start. The pressure should be greater on the upwards movement and the whole movement should be flowing and continuous.

3 Circular stroking around left and right scapulae

Stance   Walk-standing at waist level.

Hands   The main working hand is placed flat between the scapulae with the other slightly behind it. In this movement the hands circle the scapula in an upwards and outwards direction. Thus the right scapula is circled in a clockwise direction and the left in an anticlockwise direction.

The main working hand circles the scapula and remains in contact, the other hand follows but has to be lifted to pass over the main working hand at each circle. This can be done four or five times around one scapula, then the same number of times around the other scapula.

123

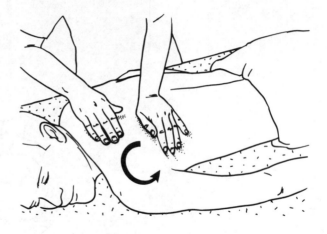

Figure 6.58 Circular stroking around left scapula

4 Figure of eight reinforced stroking around the scapulae.

Stance Walk-standing at waist level.

Hands The main working hand is placed flat between the scapulae with the other hand on top of it.

Move the hands upwards between the scapulae, around one scapula and then the other in a figure of eight. The pressure should be deeper on the upward parts of the movement.

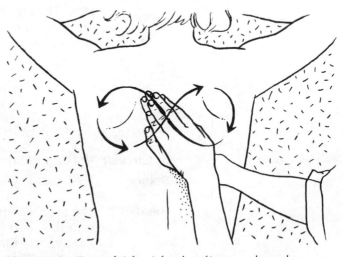

Figure 6.59 Figure of eight reinforced stroking around scapulae

---

REMEMBER

Lift the pressure when crossing bony points.

5 Flat-handed kneading

Stance Walk-standing at a level to be able to reach the whole back.

124

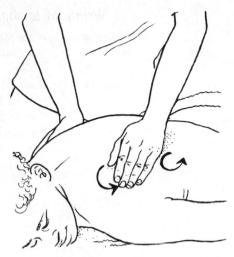

Figure 6.60   *Flat-handed kneading*

Hands   The working hand flat on the upper back with the other hand resting on the other side. Knead in circles with the hand flat on the skin moving superficial tissues on deeper tissues and only moving over the skin to shift the position of the hands. Work down one side of the body and effleurage up to start again. Repeat on other side.

6 Single-handed picking up to back of neck

Stance   Walk-standing just below shoulder level facing the head of the couch.

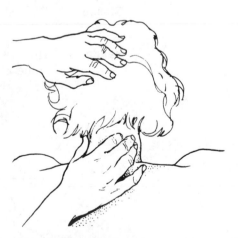

Figure 6.61   *Single-handed picking up to the back of the neck*

Hands   Working hand placed on back of neck, other hand resting on shoulder or back of the head.

With the fingers and thumb spread, pick up the muscle mass at the base of the neck, squeeze, and release. Move up to the base of the skull and down again.

125

7 Wringing to shoulders and tops of arms

Stance   Walk-standing just below shoulder level facing the head of the couch.

Hands   Both lying on the curve of the neck with fingers and thumbs spread to grasp the muscle tissue. Pick up and wring down the neck, across to the point of the shoulder and down over the upper arm. Continue picking up and move back up the arm, across to the neck, and then across the other shoulder and upper arm.

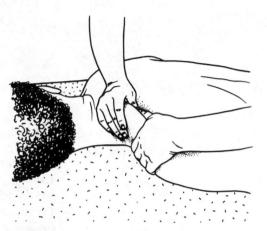

Figure 6.62 *Wringing to the shoulders and tops of arms*

8 Finger kneading/frictions at sides of spine

Stance   Walk-standing at waist level facing the head of the couch.

Hands   The tips of the middle fingers are placed on one side of the spine at the level of the base of the neck.

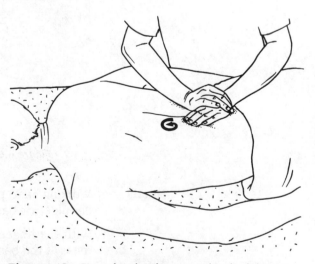

Figure 6.63 *Finger kneading/frictions at the side of the spine*

126

With the working fingers straight, feel for the slight hollows between the bony transverse processes of the vertebrae. Working downwards, knead with the finger tips in a circular direction in each hollow until the base of the spine is reached. This should only be performed once and the depth of the strokes depends on the physical state of the client. With someone young and fit the movement may be deep enough to be considered as frictions. Repeat on the other side.

9 T-shaped effleurage to the whole back

Repeat the strokes of movement 2.

10 Effleurage towards the lymph nodes

Stance   Walk-standing at a level allowing you to reach the whole length of the back.

Hands   Flat on the back at the base of the spine, one hand on each side of the spine.

In the first effleurage stroke the hands pass from the base of the back up over the back on either side of the spine to the shoulders and return to the base of the spine with a lighter pressure. The second stroke goes up the back and outwards to the axilla. The third up and out to the sides of the waist. This group of three movements may be repeated.

11 Wringing to the sides of the back

Stance   Walk-standing facing across the client.

Hands   Flat on the side of the waist furthest from the therapist. Wring down over the hip and up to the axilla. This can be repeated before moving the hands to the near side to wring in the same way.

REMEMBER

Bend the knees in order to reduce your height when working on the near side.

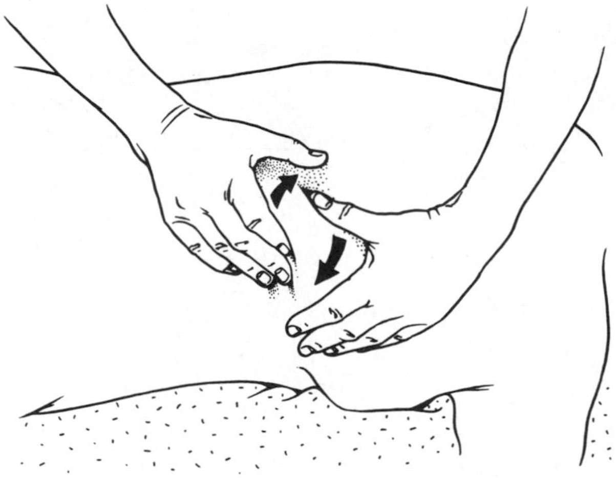

Figure 6.64 *Wringing to the sides of the back*

12 Skin rolling to the sides of the back

Stance   Walk-standing facing across the client.

Hands   Flat on the side of the back furthest from the therapist with the fingers straight and the thumbs as far away from the fingers as possible. The thumb tips should be touching.

With the flat fingers, pull the skin upwards, then push the resulting roll of skin away towards the fingers with the long surface of the thumbs. The hands travel up and down the side of the body before moving to work on the other side.

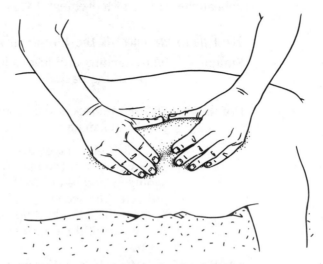

Figure 6.65   *Skin rolling to the sides of the back*

13 Transverse stroking to the lumbar region

Stance   Walk-standing facing across the client.

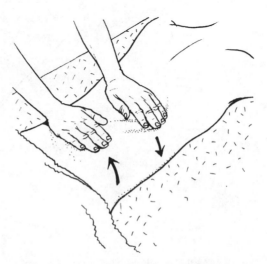

Figure 6.66   *Transverse stroking to the lumbar region*

128

Hands   Flat on the lower back.

With alternate hands, stroke across the lower back from the centre to the far side of the back, then from the centre to the near side. Repeat a number of times to cover the lumbar area.

14 Light hacking over the whole back
Stance   Stride or walk-standing facing across the back.

Hands   Relaxed with palms facing each other a little way apart and the elbows held well away from the sides.

Lightly hack up and down the whole length of the back remembering to avoid the bony points of the spine and scapula.

15 T-shaped effleurage
Repeat the strokes of movement 2. This is the last movement of the whole massage. As it is repeated, the pace gets slower and the depth lighter until the last movement finishes with the hands cupped lightly over the base of the spine. Rest the hands for a moment or two before covering the back with the towels.

Clients should be left quietly for a little while at the end of a massage, especially if the main aim of the massage is to induce relaxation. They may even be asleep. After a few minutes the client can be gently roused and asked if they want the massage medium, oil or cream removed from the skin. If so, this can be blotted off with tissue or gently wiped off with cotton wool and a good cologne or cleansing cream.

When dressed the client may be questioned as to the effectiveness of the treatment and the consultation card filled in as necessary before payment is taken and a further appointment offered.

> **REMEMBER**
> *The side of the hand is not used, only the sides of the fingers. The elbows should be well away from the sides.*

PROGRESS CHECK   Try a full body massage attempting to keep within one hour for the treatment.

Full body massage – summary

Front of legs
1 Effleurage to the sides and front of the whole of the leg.
2 Effleurage to the thigh.
3 Double-handed kneading to the thigh.
4 Single-handed kneading to the thigh.
5 Wringing to the thigh muscles.
6 Hacking to the thigh muscles.
7 Stroking around the knee.
8 Effleurage to the back of the calf with knee bent.
9 Effleurage to the lower leg.

10 Thumb kneading to the anterior tibial muscles.

11 Effleurage to the foot.

12 Kneading to the sole of the foot.

13 Single-handed hacking to the sole of the foot.

14 Thumb stroking to top of foot.

15 Thumb stroking across the sole of the foot.

16 Kneading to the toes.

17 Repeat of effleurage to the front and sides of the whole leg.

Arm massage

1 Effleurage to the posterior aspect of the arm.

2 Effleurage to the anterior aspect of the arm.

3 Single-handed picking up to the deltoid and triceps muscles.

4 Single-handed picking up to the biceps muscle

5 Wringing to the whole upper arm.

6 Light hacking to the upper arm.

7 Effleurage to the forearm.

8 Single-handed picking up to the forearm muscles.

9 Thumb stroking to the palm of the hand.

10 Thumb kneading to thenar (thumb) muscles and the hypothenar (little finger) muscles.

11 Kneading to individual fingers and thumb with stretching.

12 Thumb stroking to back of hand.

13 Circular thumb kneading to the back of the hand.

14 Repeat the effleurage to the front and back of the whole arm.

Chest massage

1 Effleurage to chest and back of neck with slight traction.

2 Stroking to one side of the neck with alternate hands.

3 Stroking to the other side of the neck with alternate hands.

4 Finger kneading to the upper fibres of the trapezius muscle from shoulders to the base of the skull.

5 Kneading to the front of the chest and shoulders.

6 Effleurage to chest and back of neck.

Abdomen

1 Effleurage to the abdomen.

2 Circular stroking to the abdomen.

3 Circular kneading over the colon.

4 Wringing to the sides and front of the abdomen.

5 Effleurage.

Back of leg

1 Effleurage to the back of the leg and buttock.
2 Effleurage to the thigh and buttock.
3 Single-handed kneading to the outer surface of the thigh.
4 Reinforced kneading to the buttock and back of thigh.
5 Wringing over the buttock and back of thigh.
6 Double-handed picking up over the hamstring muscles.
7 Hacking over buttocks and back of thigh.
8 Beating over buttocks and back of thigh.
9 Clapping over buttocks and back of thigh.
10 Effleurage to buttock and thigh.
11 Effleurage to calf.
12 Wringing to calf muscles.
13 Light hacking to calf.
14 Effleurage to back of leg and buttock

Back

1 Reverse effleurage.
2 T-shaped effleurage.
3 Circular stroking around left and right scapulae.
4 Figure of eight reinforced stroking around the scapulae.
5 Flat-handed kneading to the whole back.
6 Single-handed picking up to back of neck.
7 Wringing to shoulders and tops of arms.
8 Finger kneading/frictions at the sides of the spine.
9 T-shaped effleurage.
10 Effleurage towards lymph nodes (lower cervical, axillary and inguinal).
11 Wringing to sides of back.
12 Skin rolling to sides of back.
13 Transverse stroking to the lumbar region.
14 Light hacking over whole back.
15 T-shaped effleurage.

ACTIVITY

Start a diary to keep a record of all the massage clients you see and practise on. Note the details of their consultation and any information about their physical condition you gain during the massage.

KEY TERMS

You need to know what these words mean. Go back through the chapter or check in the glossary to find out.

Beating	Kneading	Relaxing
Clapping	Hacking	Rolling
Effleurage	Petrissage	Stimulating
Friction	Pounding	Wringing

7 Adaptations to the massage routine

After working through this chapter you will be able to:

➤ adapt the massage routine to individual areas of the body
➤ adapt the basic strokes to suit a variety of clients, thin/fat ,male/female, young/old, fit/unfit
➤ adapt a body massage for a pregnant client
➤ demonstrate massage of small children or babies
➤ adapt massage to suit a number of disabilities
➤ adapt massage to suit a slimming programme
➤ outline the principles of lymphatic drainage massage
➤ outline the principles of massage to suit clients involved in sporting activities.

Massage to individual areas of the body

When clients do not wish for a whole body massage, it is quite usual to carry out massage to individual parts of the body. Sometimes massage is carried out as part of another treatment such as foot massage during a pedicure, hand massage during a manicure or chest and neck massage as part of a facial treatment. Sometimes a client will require massage to a particular area as a treatment in itself and the commonest of these individual area massages is a back and shoulder massage for someone complaining of tension and stiffness.

Back and shoulder massage

Timing
This may be from 15 to 30 minutes depending on the client's wishes.

Position
The client can take up a position of prone lying with the clothing removed from the upper part of the body as far as the buttocks.

The massage strokes may be the same as those described for the back in the general body massage, but more time can be allotted to the area, especially those parts, usually around the scapulae, which are tense and stiff. Thus, after the figure of eight reinforced stroking, finger kneading movements around the scapulae may be performed. It is not unusual to feel 'nodules' of tension in the muscles here and in the shoulders and while it is important not to cause pain to the client, these may be worked on quite deeply. If this is the case the client should be warned of the tenderness that might be present afterwards.

It is not always necessary for the client to lie down for a back massage, particularly if the shoulder area is the important part. The client may sit

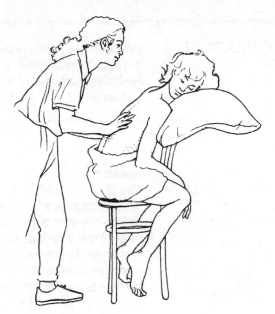

Figure 7.1 *Back massage in a sitting position*

with the head resting on a table with a pillow or cushion as a support. If treating someone at home the client may sit astride a chair using the back of the chair as a support for the head. The arms may be under the forehead or resting on the knees, whichever is most comfortable.

There are specific supports on the market (see p. 10, Chapter 2) which can be placed on a table or couch for the client to rest on. These are also convenient to use if you are visiting clients in the home or office.

When the client is sitting, it is not an easy position for the therapist and it takes a little practice to be effective. It is only suitable for a short massage as the lower half of the back cannot be effectively worked on.

SUGGESTED ROUTINE for back and shoulder massage if the client is in prone lying.

1 Effleurage to upper back and shoulders and tops of arms.
2 Circular stroking around right and left scapulae.
3 Figure of eight reinforced stroking around scapulae.
4 Flat-handed kneading over upper back and shoulders.
5 Single-handed picking up to back of neck.
6 Wringing across shoulders and tops of arms.
7 Finger kneading/frictions at sides of the spine.
8 Finger kneading/frictions around right and left scapulae.
9 Light hacking across shoulders.
10 Effleurage to the upper back and shoulders and tops of arms.

Foot and leg massage

This is often suggested for a client with tired feet or tired, 'puffy' legs. For instance for a client who does a lot of standing rather than walking during the working day. (For lymphatic drainage massage, see p. 142.)

133

SAFE PRACTICE ▷ *Remember the contra-indications to massage that might cause swelling of a limb — thrombosis, phlebitis or severe varicose veins. If in doubt, refer the client to their medical advisor and never massage over tender or swollen areas when the cause is unknown.*

Position

The client should be lying and it will help the massage to be effective if the legs can be slightly elevated. This elevation can be achieved either by raising the end of the couch or by placing pillows under the whole length of the legs. The legs must not be raised more than about 25 degrees. At this angle lymphatic drainage can occur freely to the inguinal lymph nodes and massage is easy to apply. The legs should never be raised so high as to make the massage awkward for the therapist.

Preparation

The soles of the feet should be lightly wiped with cologne to remove any dirt or perspiration. The leg not being worked on should be covered with a towel.

SUGGESTED ROUTINE for foot and leg massage. (The numbers of repetitions of each stroke depends on time available.)

1 Effleurage to the sides of the leg starting at the toes and ending at the inguinal nodes.
2 Effleurage to the sides of the lower leg and front of thigh.
3 Effleurage to sides of lower leg and back of thigh.
4 Double-handed circular kneading to the thigh.
5 Wringing to the thigh muscles.
6 Hacking to the thigh muscles.
7 Light beating or pounding to the thigh muscles.
8 Effleurage to the thigh.
9 Stroking around the knee.
10 Effleurage to the lower leg directed to the back of the knee.
11 With the leg rolled outwards, wringing to the calf muscles.
12 Effleurage to the lower leg.
13 Effleurage to the sole of the foot.
14 Kneading to sole of the foot.
15 Single-handed hacking to sole of the foot.
16 Thumb stroking to top of the foot.
17 Thumb stroking across sole of the foot.
18 Kneading with gentle traction to individual toes.
19 Effleurage to whole leg.

The movements described for the hands and feet may be used on their own for a client who is bed bound, for example a hospitalised patient.

From the whole body massage routine select movements suitable to make up:

a a hand massage routine

b a foot massage routine.

Carry out one of each.

Adapting massage to various clients

Adaptations to general massage to accommodate clients of different age groups, sizes and physical and mental states

The initial consultation procedure should elicit information useful for selecting massage movements and methods to suit individual clients. Information such as age, lifestyle and medical history can be gained in this way, but it is only when starting to massage that many physical characteristics are noted.

Client preference as to depth of massage should be obtained by direct questioning during the first treatment and noted on the treatment card for future reference. Often a client needs to be encouraged to give direction in this. It is not enough to ask, 'Is that all right?' or to say, 'Tell me if it is too deep'. The client needs to be told that it will help you if they can give a definite indication as to how firm they like the massage.

The muscle tone of a client can be felt when massage is being performed on the larger muscle groups and in general muscle tone is better in younger, fitter clients than in older ones. If muscle tone is poor then care must be taken with the petrissage and percussion movements so that the muscles are not compressed too hard against bone or over-stretched during wringing or rolling techniques. Similar care must be taken with very thin clients, young or old, as deep massage over bony points will be very uncomfortable.

An obese client presents different problems. The muscle tone often cannot be easily assessed due to overlying fatty tissue and there may be a temptation to think that the density of the tissue means that it is insensitive. It is not unusual for an obese client to complain that massage is painful over areas such as the thighs. Client feedback must be obtained and noted.

GOOD PRACTICE ▷ *When working on clients, male or female, care must be taken to protect the client's modesty by draping towels to cover parts not being treated. This is to protect the therapist as well as the client. Therapists should be aware of the dangers of working with clients of the opposite sex unchaperoned and should take care not to leave themselves open to accusations of unprofessional behaviour.*

A female therapist should avoid the abdominal area of a male client.

A male therapist should avoid the chest/breast and abdominal areas of a female client.

In general terms the male body is firmer than the female, although this depends on their fitness and exercise regime. Women have a layer of fat under the skin which softens the line of the female body, hiding the muscle outlines and making the body softer to handle.

The male body may be hairy which makes massage difficult. Hairy chests and legs are common but backs and arms can also be very hairy. If the body is hairy then the massage must be adapted to avoid working against the lie of the hair.

* Use more oil or talc than usual to allow free movement of hands.
* Effleurage or stroking should be performed in the direction of the hair.
* When using petrissage take care not to pull on the hair.

Clients book massage treatments for different reasons; for relaxation, for stimulation or alongside a slimming/fitness regime and this will also affect the type of massage given.

It should also be noted that many clients will be nervous at their initial treatment and it is the therapist's responsibility to put them at ease. An atmosphere of quiet and reassurance that professional standards are maintained is essential.

ACTIVITY

Try to select as wide a variety of clients as possible and in your massage diary note adaptations appropriate to age differences, size, fitness, etc.

Massage for the pregnant client

You should ask a pregnant client to check with her medical advisor whether there is any reason why she should not have massage.

SAFE PRACTICE

Remember that massage over the abdomen is contra-indicated during the first three months of a pregnancy.

Pregnant women often benefit from massage because they tend to tire more easily. Their posture alters as their figure shape changes, causing stress on the lower back and legs, and their weight increases causing tired legs and feet. Pregnant women often find sleep difficult and the relaxing effects of massage can help this insomnia.

The body massage routine may be used with a number of adaptations.

* Omit any percussion/tapotement movements.
* All the movements should be smooth and gentle.
* The positioning of the client will need to be altered as she will be unable to lie on her stomach. To massage the back and back of the legs she can lie in the recovery position or on her side with supporting pillows under the upper leg and arm. When she lies on her back, put a

136

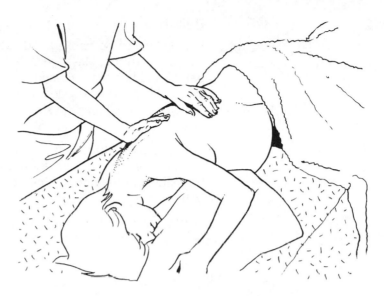

Figure 7.2 *Positioning a pregnant client for massage to the back/back of legs*

small cushion under her knees to relax the abdomen and flatten the lower back.

The only movements that may be done over the abdomen (after three months) are stroking movements.

1 Stroke around the abdomen clockwise, using both hands, one following the other in a gentle, flowing movement.

2 Stroke up the centre of the abdomen very gently and then very lightly down the sides.

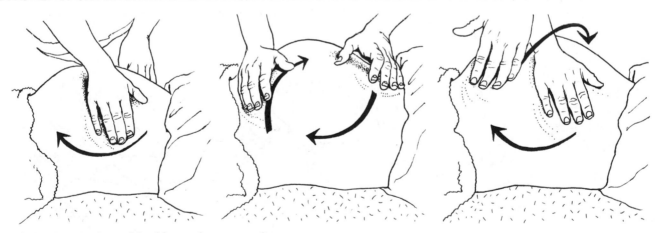

Figure 7.3 *Stroking on the abdomen of a pregnant client*

Children and babies

These are unlikely to be clients in a salon, but parents who benefit from massage will often ask how they can massage their children and you may find it a good idea to hold occasional classes for parents. Parents should be warned that children love to be massaged and they could find themselves still being asked for a massage when their children are grown up!

Babies

Babies love to be stroked and caressed and a loving touch is a natural part of parenting. Massage is just an extension of this which will benefit parent and baby by helping in the bonding process. In many parts of the world babies are massaged and rubbed from birth, sometimes even with the aim of moulding the shape of the head and body after a difficult birth.

Massage can help to calm a fractious baby and is of special benefit to parents who find they have a baby who is reluctant to sleep. It can calm the baby and the parent. The best time of day is just before or after the baby's bath.

A tiny baby can be massaged lying along the parents knees or on the changing table or floor.

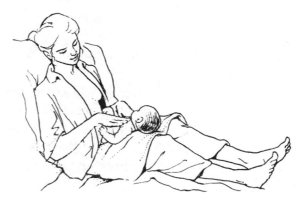

Figure 7.4   *Massaging a baby lying along the knees*

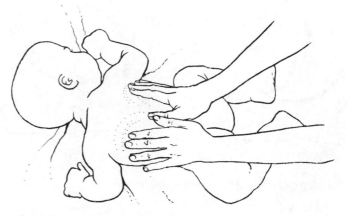

Figure 7.5   *Massaging a baby on a table or floor*

The massage medium should be a good quality vegetable oil, such as grapeseed or almond oil, but preferably not baby oil as that is a mineral oil. Talc is not suitable as the powder may be inhaled by the baby.

There is no need for a rigid or special sequence, the movements are nearly all stroking movements except for gentle squeezing and wringing with the fingertips on the limbs and back if the baby seems to enjoy it. It is usual to start on the front of the baby's body so that they can see the parent.

The face can be included with gentle thumb stroking across the forehead centre to the sides and around the nose and chin.

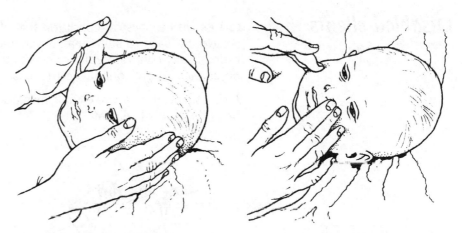

Figure 7.6 *Massaging a baby's face*

Very often the parents just require the confidence to try and a class with other parents is just the place to start.

Children

In the same way, clients who come for massage and express an interest can be encouraged to massage their children. Children of all ages enjoy it and respond well to relaxing strokes. It need not be a formal massage session, just some of the effleurage and petrissage strokes need be used that are used on adults, but applied more lightly and for less time.

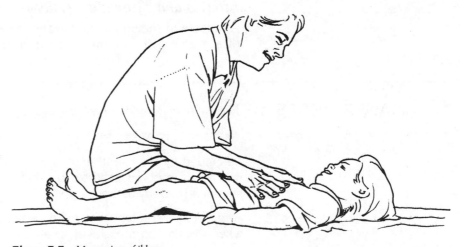

Figure 7.7 *Massaging children*

If a child becomes restless, that is the time to stop. There is often no need for the child to undress and have oil on the skin, massage can take place through light clothing and be part of a play session.

Disabled clients

Clients with a physical condition that affects movement can usually receive massage to suit them. A variable height couch which is hydraulically controlled allows clients to reach the couch and then be raised to a height to suit the therapist.

A client who uses a wheelchair may transfer to a couch or prefer to be treated in the wheelchair.

— REMEMBER —

Many wheelchair users are extremely fit people apart from being unable to walk and often take part in sports ranging from archery to a very fast handball. Be careful not to seem patronising.

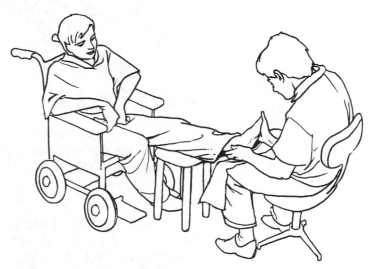

Figure 7.8 *Massaging a disabled client*

Arthritis and rheumatic conditions

Arthritis and rheumatic conditions sometimes limit clients' mobility and often cause pain in joints and the surrounding muscles.

SAFE PRACTICE ▷ *Remember that working over hot swollen joints is contra-indicated.*

Be guided by the client as to what position they can adopt. Then the massage can be adapted to suit that position. Pillows can be placed to support the body as necessary.

Avoid percussion/tapotement movements and be guided by the client when working on muscles near affected joints. Never work over painful areas.

REMEMBER

The client must give their written permission to the doctor before medical details can be released.

If a request for treatment is made by someone with a neurological condition such as multiple sclerosis (MS) or by someone who has had a stroke or other serious illness, always consult their doctor.

You might find that you can work in conjunction with other therapists, perhaps with their physiotherapist to the advantage of you both. The physiotherapist will probably be concentrating on rehabilitation and maintaining normal movement and might welcome the assistance of someone who can help relieve general symptoms of tension.

Massage as part of a slimming regime

Therapists specialising in body massage are employed in salons and centres which specialise in weight control programmes. This is not because massage makes clients lose weight, but because they benefit in other ways which are helpful to their particular regime.

A typical client visiting a health or fitness centre will, after a full consultation and possibly a medical check-up, be given advice on an exercise and diet regime aimed at achieving a weight loss of not more than 2 lb (less than 1 kg) per week.

There are of course many treatments offered by beauty salons which aim to improve and help to reshape the figure alongside diet and exercise.

The role of massage in this field is different. Massage can help motivate a client to stick to the diet and exercise regime. It can help clients' self image and their consciousness of the state of their body. The touch and attention of the therapist makes them more aware of their posture and stance, important factors in looking good. It can also help clients who have a distorted idea of their size as it often is the case that slimmers think themselves plumper than they are.

The more direct effects are the stimulation of the circulation to the skin and subcutaneous tissues, improving the texture and look of the skin.

A common complaint sometimes, but not always, associated with overweight is localised deposits of fatty tissue which do not easily respond to diet. This condition is known in the beauty business as cellulite and should not be confused with cellulitis which is a medical condition of inflammation of the tissues and like all inflammatory conditions is a contra-indication to massage.

Cellulite tends to occur mainly in women and appears on the waist and hips, buttocks and thighs, inner knee, upper arm and the upper back. It often looks lumpy and dimples on pressure and will frequently feel colder to the touch than surrounding tissue.

REMEMBER

Always check with the client, fatty tissue and particularly cellulite is often much more sensitive than you might think.

A body massage is adapted for a client who is overweight or who has cellulite by spending more time on the areas worst affected. Stimulating movements such as pounding and hacking should be included to soften hard, fatty areas and stimulate local circulation. The effleurage and petrissage movements can be made firmer and brisker to stimulate the lymphatic and general circulatory systems.

Massage to stimulate lymphatic drainage

ACTIVITY

Make sure you understand the arrangement of the lymphatic vessels and nodes. Check the direction of lymphatic drainage (see Figures 4.11 and 4.12).

All massage will stimulate the lymphatic drainage to some extent but occasionally a specific part of the body, usually the legs, will benefit from more specific massage aimed to reduce water retention and puffiness.

* Always remove any restrictive clothing.
* If possible elevate the part to be treated for a time (10–30 minutes) before the massage.
* Elevate the limb or part no more than 45 degrees during the massage.
* Always work on the most proximal part first, working down the limb a handbreadth at a time.
* Think of the limb as a four-sided tube to be emptied and work with hands on opposite sides so that first a movement is performed thoroughly with the hands on the top and bottom surfaces of the limb then on opposite sides.

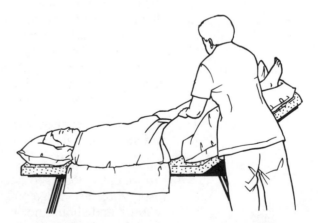

Figure 7.9 *Elevating the legs to assist lymphatic drainage*

* Start each movement lightly, slowly getting deeper as the area softens.
* Massage strokes that are appropriate are
  a to soften the area
  slow, double-handed kneading, compressing the limb gently between the hands
  slow, gentle picking up.
  b to drain the area single-handed vibrations, with the other hand giving counter pressure
  effleurage towards the nearest lymph nodes.

* On small parts, such as the ankle and foot, thumb kneading and stroking should be used.
* When the limb has been treated section by section, effleurage to the whole limb may be used to end the massage.

SAFE PRACTICE ▷ *Massage for a client with the condition known as lymphoedema should not be undertaken without checking that massage is not contra-indicated. Lymphoedema is a condition where the lymphatic drainage is no longer effective in draining the limb concerned, it may be a result of lifesaving treatment for cancer which has destroyed lymph nodes or may occur for unknown reasons. The limb affected will be very swollen and hard and care must be taken not to damage the skin which can be vulnerable to infection.*

If massage is to be applied to a limb affected by lymphoedema, then the massage must be gentle and superficial as deep rough movements may damage the tissues and increase the swelling. The strokes must always be in the direction of lymphatic drainage and towards unaffected areas.

Sports massage

There has been a resurgence of interest in massage as an aid to athletes in the last decade. With many more people becoming concerned about health and fitness, they are taking a much more active part in sports often as very keen amateurs. This increased participation has led to a demand for ways to improve performance and the part-time sportsman today may be as competitive as a professional may have been a few years ago. As training builds up progressively a point can be reached where the body is no longer able to recover fully between sessions and performance will level off or even decline. At this stage the body is vulnerable to injury if changes in the regime are not made. Massage can be used for the general relaxation of the muscles as well as helping specific problem areas to improve the condition of muscles and help prevent injury. Manual massage has a long tradition in many countries and athletes in the past used to take advantage of this treatment long before physiotherapists and osteopaths existed. Many modern sportsmen and women have become excellent massage therapists because they have a real understanding of the anatomy and physiology necessary and of the sports concerned.

Uses of massage in sport

* General treatment to maintain muscles in good condition by increasing the circulation in the muscles.
* Pre-event to prepare muscles for strenuous work.
* Post-event to restore muscles after strenuous work.
* To treat local areas which show incomplete recovery from injury.

General treatment

Ideally a competitive sportsman will have massage at least once a week, preferably after the hardest training session of the week and it should always be followed by one or two days of lighter training. When massage is given once a week it must be deep and thorough whereas if done more often it can be lighter. Massage should be more frequent at the beginning of the training season than at the end.

As the aim of this massage is relaxation and improvement of the circulation to muscles, the routine can follow the general directions for body massage using the same type of strokes.

* Effleurage and stroking movements can be used especially to feel for tension in particular muscles. Deep stroking movements can be applied to individual muscles along the length of the muscle fibres.
* Petrissage movements should start superficially and increase in depth as superficial muscles relax.
* Tapotement/percussion movements should not be too heavy or sharp just because the muscles look so firm.

Vibrations and shakings are particularly useful in treating tense muscles.

* A vibration movement can be applied using the hand or the fingers depending on the size of the area being treated and when applied with gentle pressure is very relaxing.
* Shaking movements are applied by using one or both hands to grasp the muscle and shake it from side to side and is useful after deeper movements which may have caused discomfort and tension.
* Friction can be used to warm an area before other massage movements.

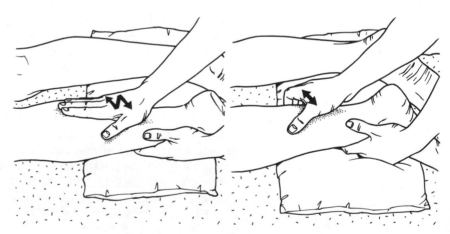

Figure 7.10 *Vibration*   **Figure 7.11** *Shaking*

* Frictions, applied with the pads of the thumb or fingers, are used on problem areas such as scar tissue or hard bands of muscle which develop as a result of overuse and injury. The frictions will increase local circulation and soften adhesions in the muscle. They should only be used by an experienced sports therapist.

The main adaptations of massage movements when working on sportsmen and women are to depth and direction. Because of the level of muscle tone and fitness, all movements may be used to a greater depth. Direction is varied according to the effects required. If stimulation of the circulation is needed then the direction of the strokes will be as usual, but if stretching the muscles is required then the direction of the muscle fibres must be known and understood.

The hands may be used differently. Whereas in a routine massage the palm of the hand will be in contact for the majority of movements, in a sports massage the thumbs, fingers, heel of the hand and even the elbow may be used to obtain the necessary depth and to concentrate the pressure on a specific area.

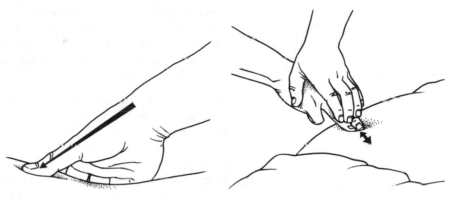

Figure 7.12   *Using the thumb*   **Figure 7.13**   *Using deep friction*

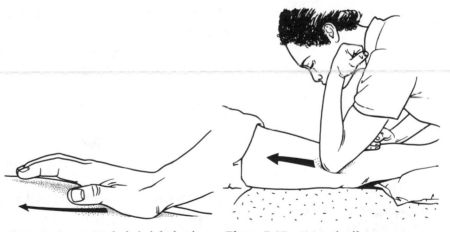

Figure 7.14   *Using the heel of the hand*   **Figure 7.15**   *Using the elbow*

PROGRESS CHECK   Try out all the techniques shown on a client who is fit and has very firm muscles.

Pre-event massage

Only light massage should be given before an event. No deep massage movements should be used for four or five days before a competition or important training session. It has been shown that some heavy massage strokes, especially percussion, produce an immediate decrease in muscle performance and an increase of creatine kinase in the blood suggesting muscle damage.

Post-event massage

The purpose of massage after exercise is to help the removal of the waste products of the activity from the muscles and the sooner this is carried out the better. If the athlete waits too long then the muscles to be worked on may be stiff and sore, making the massage much more uncomfortable. The rate of work should be slow with the depth increasing gradually as superficial muscles relax.

Avoid all percussion movements

To treat local areas which show incomplete recovery from injury

This is usually work undertaken by specialised therapists with a medical background such as osteopaths and chartered physiotherapists, but massage therapists might well find themselves working with such staff to the benefit of both. Acute sporting injuries should never be treated by unqualified personnel.

Muscle stretching is an important part of the athlete's fitness regime and exercises will be devised to stretch individual and groups of muscles. When a muscle is stretched along its length as in exercise, the fibres are drawn closer together. Massage can stretch a muscle in any direction and so can be used to separate bundles of muscle fibres by working across them. Deep frictions applied across the muscle fibres can also be used to soften deep scar tissue which may be present in soft tissue as a result of old injuries.

Differences between sports massage and the more usual types of massage

* The massage is being performed on people who know a great deal about their bodies and to whom even a minor degree of malfunction is noticeable.
* The bodies being treated are very fit, strong and hard.
* Effleurage is used to a much lesser extent; it is often diagnostic as the therapist feels for problems.
* Most movements are on specific muscles or muscle groups, superficial and deep.
* Knowledge of the musculo-skeletal structure of the area is very important.
* Knowledge of the muscles used in specific sports or activities is an advantage.

Points to be considered in treating athletes

* Use a couch which is firm and strong, preferably one where the height can be altered as you will need to exert a greater degree of force than usual.
* Posture and stance should enable the therapist to exert pressure where needed – work close to the couch and use your body weight.
* To reach deeper muscles you need to work through superficial muscles and connective tissue. To avoid the superficial muscles tensing up, start gently and instead of working directly on tender spots, approach from different angles.

REMEMBER

Many disabled people are fine athletes too.

146

* Even though problems may be present in one area they may be caused by or cause problems in another, e.g. if the problem is in the foot treat the whole leg and look at the lower back, if in the shoulder, check the neck region.

ACTIVITY	Make a list of five sports that friends participate in. Work out the main muscle groups that are likely to be used most often in these sports and list how you would alter your usual massage routine to treat a person who participates in each.

8 Essential oils for aromatherapy massage

After working through this chapter you will be able to:
➤ define an essential oil
➤ outline the factors governing the quality of essential oils
➤ describe the effects of the main chemical categories of essential oils
➤ describe the main qualities of a selected number of essential oils
➤ describe the qualities of a number of carrier oils
➤ select the amounts of carrier and essential oil for massage
➤ carry out a consultation for an aromatherapy massage
➤ prepare a plan for an aromatherapy massage
➤ select oils which blend together well for aromatherapy massage.

Aromatherapy is the name given to treatments that use essential oils – the pure, volatile portions of aromatic plant products. There has been a huge surge of interest in such treatments as part of the growing regard for holistic therapies and complementary medicine. There are many books and courses now for anyone interested in becoming an aromatherapist; beauty therapists, massage therapists and medical personnel such as nurses, occupational therapists and chartered physiotherapists are all becoming involved. It is a subject which can be studied to many levels, so that some people will call themselves aromatherapists who have only a limited knowledge of oils and others will have studied and practised for many years. As more people become aware of the benefits of aromatherapy, training standards will be raised and the levels standardised with a full qualification necessary to practise.

These chapters are meant to provide a starting point for the beginner and to provide a basis for future development. As with other therapies, learning must start somewhere but should never stop. Aromatherapy becomes more fascinating the more you learn.

ACTIVITY

Re-read Chapter 4 with particular reference to aromatherapy, noting references in the sections on the permeability of the skin, sensitisation and allergy and on the nervous system and olfactory receptors.

Because essential oils are said to be good for physical and mental conditions there is a temptation for the practitioner to regard aromatherapy as a form of medicine. If that were so, then beauty

148

therapists and those without some medical training would not be using it. Aromatherapy is the use of essential oils to help maintain people in good health and to improve their well being. Clients with medical conditions should always be referred to their doctor.

Essential oils

Essential oils are aromatic substances present at very low concentrations in different parts of plants; in leaves, flower petals, berries and even twigs. When they are extracted from plants and bottled as pure essential oils, their concentration is 100%. They are available for purchase in this form by the general public as well as aromatherapists and should always be adequately diluted for safe use.

Extraction

Oils are extracted from plants by several different methods.

Expression

A few essential oils, such as the citrus oils where the oil is contained in the outer part of the skin, can be obtained by simple pressure. (Examples: lemon, orange, bergamot.)

Distillation

Some essential oils are obtained by distillation. The plant parts are heated in water or steam and the vapour given off is cooled to produce a liquid which is a mixture of essential oil and water. The essential oil can then be easily separated and drawn off to leave perfumed water behind as a by-product.

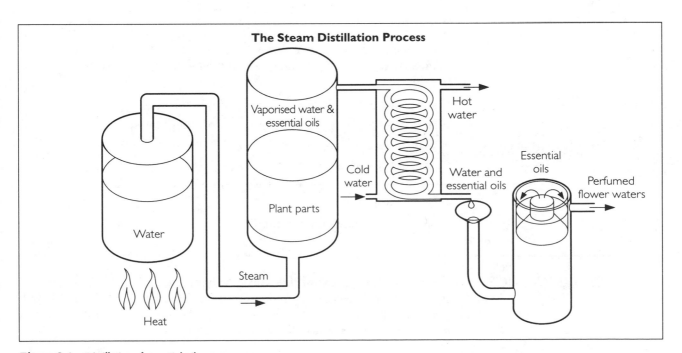

Figure 8.1 *Distillation of essential oils*

Solvent extraction

Solvent extraction is a method used to obtain some floral oils. The plants are immersed in hydrocarbon solvents to dissolve the essential oils. The solution is then distilled to leave behind a mixture of wax and oil known as a 'concrete'. The wax can then be dissolved in alcohol which in turn can be evaporated off leaving an 'absolute'. Absolutes differ from true essential oils in that they are generally thicker and more viscous. They are more often used in perfumery than in aromatherapy.

More recently carbon dioxide has been used as a solvent to extract essential oils successfully. By using carbon dioxide in a state known as 'hypercritical' at high pressure, it becomes a very effective solvent which does not contaminate the oils. This method requires bulky and expensive equipment but the number of essential oils extracted by this method that are commercially available is increasing.

Enfleurage

Enfleurage is a traditional method of extraction that is only used today for some very expensive oils such as rose and jasmine. It involves spreading the petals of the plant on fat or oil which absorbs the essence and then extracting it from the fat by using solvents to separate them. However even rose and jasmine these days are mostly extracted by the more commercial solvent or distillation methods.

Quality

The quality of essential oils is most important and care must be taken to use only oils which are pure and unadulterated. The best advice when starting is to deal only with a reputable supplier who is known to stock oils of the highest quality. Good suppliers are also the best source of advice on which oils to order, for example there are a number of different oils called lavender each with its own qualities and a good supplier will be able to advise you of the differences.

All plants have a common English name and a recognised scientific Latin name which identifies it more accurately and it is wise to become familiar with the Latin name to avoid mistakes when ordering and using the oils.

Factors which can affect the quality of oils include:

* choice of the best possible member of the plant species
* where the plant was grown
* whether it was grown organically
* how it was harvested and at what time of day
* what method of extraction was used
* how the oils have been stored.

SAFE PRACTICE ▷ *Once the oils are purchased they should be kept away from the light in dark, tightly-stoppered glass bottles to preserve them. For safety's sake the bottles used should not be open topped, but should have some form of drop dispenser in the neck and of course be kept out of the reach of children.*

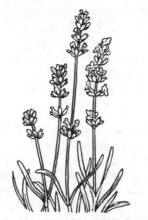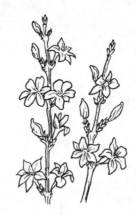

Figure 8.2 *Lavender and jasmine*

Categories of oils

There are a number of ways of classifying oils

1 By their volatility rate – that is how quickly they evaporate into the air.

Top notes evaporate the fastest, act quickly and tend to be stimulating. Examples: lemon and other citrus oils.

Middle notes evaporate more slowly and are most often used to help the general metabolism. Examples: geranium and other floral and fruity oils.

Base notes evaporate slowly and are relaxing and sedating. Example: sandalwood.

Some therapists will take this into account when mixing a blend of oils, using a base note oil to hold and 'fix' a top note oil. If you smell a mixture of oils containing different 'notes', you will smell the top notes first followed by the middle and base notes.

2 By the eastern yin and yang philosophy. The terms yin and yang are descriptions of opposite 'energies' or qualities. Yin describes cool, moist, calming, feminine qualities (e.g. rose, geranium), whereas yang describes hot, dry, stimulating, masculine qualities (e.g. juniper). Many oils fall between these extremes and the nearer they are to the middle the more 'balancing' they will be (e.g. sandalwood). Some therapists take this into account when selecting oils for a particular client and when deciding what effects they need to produce – calming, balancing or stimulating.

3 By the chemical constituents of the oils. This is a much more complex matter as each essential oil will consist of many chemical components which may even vary in oils of the same name depending on where the plant was grown and under what conditions.

Oils contain chemicals in varying proportions and tend to be classified according to which of the chemicals is predominant. These chemicals can be put in place on a chart according to their general yin or yang qualities. The chemicals also have general effects which can be described. Table 8.1 summarises the effects of certain chemicals and shows their relation to the yin and yang qualities.

YIN (calming)

Aldehydes – anti-inflammatory, antiseptic, anti-rheumatic, very calming and soothing.

Ketones – healing, good for skin and scars, sedative, loosens mucous and softens fat so often used for people with bronchitis and cellulite. **(Ketones should not be used for too long or in high concentrations when they may be toxic.)**

Esters – the most widespread group of chemicals found in essential oils; anti-spasmodic, anti-inflammatory, anti-parasitic, cooling and soothing.

Ethers – anti-inflammatory, anti spasmodic and anti-stress.

Sesquiterpenes – anti inflammatory, anti-allergic, anti-parasitic; good for people with heart conditions and asthma

_____ Balancing line _____

Sesquialcohols – act as a general tonic.

Alcohols – germicidal; some are very stimulating, but others are much less so.

Terpenes – antiseptic and anti inflammatory; they can help to improve the blood and lymphatic circulation.

Oxides – expectorant and decongestant, helping people to cough. Some are anti-parasitic, anti-viral and antiseptic.

Phenols – anti-bacterial, anti-viral, anti-fungal and anti-parasitic. **(Oils in the phenol category are very stimulating and are never used in aromatherapy massage.)**

YANG (stimulating)

Table 8.1 *The properties of essential oils*

Selection of oils for use

Selection of oils for use with a particular client is the most important part of aromatherapy and can be very daunting for the beginner.

When starting, select from a limited list, 8–10 oils should be enough, growing to 15–20 as experience increases. In the selection you choose include more calming and balancing oils than stimulating oils, select the more commonly used oils and be guided by a good supplier. Make sure you know if any of the oils have any contra-indications or can have harmful effects.

A possible list might include the following oils. The oils are listed alphabetically along with their Latin names, predominant chemical category, their best known effects and some of the oils that can be used with them to make a good blend.

Yin oils

Basil (*Ocimum basilicum*) – top note, ether.
* Steadying, good for nervous clients, good for muscle aches and pains and for coughs and colds.
* Blends well with bergamot, geranium.

SAFE PRACTICE ▷ * Not to be used during pregnancy.

Bergamot (*Citrus aurantium bergamia*) – top note, ester.
* Uplifting; good for people who are anxious or depressed and having difficulty sleeping.
* Blends well with lavender, neroli, basil.

SAFE PRACTICE ▷ * Bergamot has been shown to sensitise skin to ultra-violet so do not use within three hours of going out into the sun or using a sun-bed.
* Bergamot should not be used on children.

Clary sage (*Salvia sclarea*) – middle to base note, ester.
* Good for exhaustion and overwork, a good muscle relaxant, anti-depressant.
* Blends well with citrus oils, frankincense, geranium, juniper.

SAFE PRACTICE ▷ * Not to be used during pregnancy or the menopause.

Chamomile (*Matricaria chamomilla*) – middle note, sesquiterpene.
* Soothing; a very gentle oil, good on the skin, very calming and good for people suffering from tension, anxiety and related conditions.
* Blends well with lavender, patchouli, geranium, benzoin.

Lavender (*Lavendula augustofolia*) – middle note, ester.
* Boosts the immune system, calming, balancing, healing (especially burns), muscular pain, problem skins. The most versatile and useful oil.
* Blends well with other oils especially floral and citrus oils.

Lemon grass (*Cymbopogon citratus*) – top note, aldehyde.
* Strengthening; good for muscle aches and pains, stomach upsets.
* Blends well with geranium, lavender.

SAFE PRACTICE ▷ * Not to be used on children.

Peppermint (*Mentha piperita*) – top to middle note, ketone.

* Cooling; traditionally used for stomach upsets, also for clearing the head and for coughs and colds. Very good for tired feet.
* Blends well with benzoin, rosemary.

SAFE PRACTICE ▷

* *Can irritate sensitive skins.*
* *Avoid during the first four months of pregnancy.*

Petitgrain (*Citrus aurantium*) – top note, ester

* Anti-stress, good for oily skins and stomach upsets.
* Blends well with rosemary, lavender, geranium, bergamot, clary sage.

Rose geranium (*Pelargonium graveolens*) – middle note, alcohol/ester.

* Balancing; good for dry and red skins, it stimulates the lymphatic system and can be used for cellulite.
* Blends well with most oils, especially citrus oils, lavender, bergamot and basil.

Rosemary (*Rosemarinus officianalis*) – middle note, ketone.

* Uplifting – after lavender, the most commonly used oil. It is useful for people with colds or other respiratory problems. Good for stiffness and discomfort in the muscles.
* Blends well with basil, citrus oils, frankincense, peppermint.

SAFE PRACTICE ▷

* *Rosemary is contra-indicated in pregnant or epileptic clients and in those with high blood pressure.*
* *Rosemary should not be used for too long a period as it can be stimulating.*

Yang oils

Black pepper (*Piper nigrum*) – middle note, terpene.

* Stimulating, good for the circulation and conditions related to poor circulation. Can stimulate the appetite.
* Blends well with frankincense, sandalwood.

Eucalyptus (*Eucalyptus globulus or radiata*) – top note, oxide.

* Decongestant helping people with colds or bronchitis to cough. Also relieves muscular or rheumatic pain.
* Blends well with benzoin, lavender, pine.

Frankincense (*Boswellia carteri*) – base note, terpene.

* Rejuvenating, very good on older skins, good for chest conditions – especially stress-related ones.
* Blends well with basil, black pepper, citrus oils, lavender, sandalwood.

Juniper (*Juniperus communis*) – middle note, terpene

* Diuretic, good for people with fluid retention or cellulite and can be helpful in cases of cystitis. Good on some problem skins, e.g. acne. Can be used as a disinfectant.
* Blends well with benzoin, lavender, sandalwood.

Lemon (*Citrus limon*) – top note, terpene

* Useful for clients recovering from viral-type illnesses. Also stimulates the circulation, so useful over areas of fat and cellulite and in rheumatic conditions. Refreshing.
* Blends well with lavender, neroli, ylang ylang.

SAFE PRACTICE ▷
* *Can cause skin irritation, so needs to be used in very low dosage.*
* *Do not use during pregnancy.*

Rosewood (*Aniba roseadora*) – middle note, alcohol.

* Gentle, very good for skin and stress-related conditions.
* Blends well with most oils, especially citrus and floral oils.

Sandalwood (*Santalum album*) – base note, sesquialcohol.

* Balancing; good on the skin and for stress-related conditions and nervous tension.
* Blends well with lavender, black pepper, bergamot, geranium.

Tea tree (*Melaleuca alternifolia*) – top note, alcohol.

* One of the best known of the essential oils and now being incorporated into creams and soaps for its anti-fungal, anti-bacterial and anti-viral qualities. Particularly useful in helping fungal conditions such as thrush and athlete's foot. It seems to stimulate the immune system and is particularly valuable if a cold or flu might be developing.
* Blends well with lavender, rosemary, clary sage.

Ylang ylang (*Cananga odorata*) – base note, sesquialcohol.

* Warming; soothes and boosts confidence, traditionally known as an aphrodisiac.
* Blends well with rosewood, bergamot.

Oils such as rose, melissa and jasmine are much too expensive to include in a starting list.

SAFE PRACTICE ▷ *Note that some of these oils are contra-indicated during pregnancy. Until fully qualified it is wise to avoid using essential oils to treat children and women who are pregnant or breast feeding.*

Carrier oils

Essential oils are very concentrated and should never be used undiluted on the skin. For an aromatherapy massage they must be mixed with a carrier oil which will provide lubrication for the massage as well as carrying the therapeutic essential oils being used.

Although mineral oils such as baby oil are sometimes used for massage they are not suitable as a carrier oils as they are not easily absorbed by the skin. You can use any vegetable oil so long as it is fairly light and does not have a strong smell which would overpower the essential oils. Just as a good cook will insist that the olive oil they use should be of the finest quality, so an aromatherapist will use only carrier oils that are organically grown, unrefined and cold pressed. Again, the advice of a reputable supplier is invaluable.

The carrier oil chosen can be used on its own with the essential oils or can have small amounts of other oils mixed with them. When beginning to mix oils, grapeseed oil is probably best used as a carrier oil as it is easily available and not expensive. Sweet almond oil is also an excellent choice. Other oils may be mixed with the carrier oils in small amounts before blending in the essential oils.

Examples are:

* Wheatgerm oil which is an anti-oxidant and so acts to prevent other oils going rancid. It contains vitamin E and is very good for scarred skin.
* Avocado oil which is rich and nourishing. It is especially good for dry or ageing skin, as is peach kernel and apricot kernel oil.
* Evening primrose oil which is a rich source of gamma linoleic acid and beneficial vitamins.

If any of these oils are to be used they are usually added to the carrier oil in the proportion of 10% to 90% main carrier.

All vegetable carrier oils will go off and become rancid eventually and will become unfit for use. They should be kept cool and not mixed with essential oils until ready for use.

Mixing the oils for aromatherapy massage

To prepare a blend for massage you will need:

* A glass or clear plastic measuring bottle that is marked in millilitres.
* A glass rod for stirring.

The amount of carrier oil needed for the massage is measured into the

156

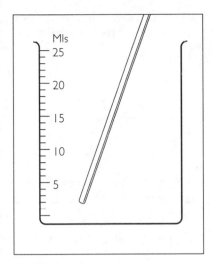

Figure 8.3 *Mixing equipment*

bottle and the drops of essential oils added. It is then stirred with the glass rod or shaken if there is a stopper, and then it is ready for use.

Amounts of oil needed for massage will vary but a useful 'rule of thumb' is: for a full body massage allow 10 ml for a small person, 14 ml for a medium size and up to 20 ml for a large person. In women, the dress size is a good indicator.

Try not to mix too much oil as it will be wasted

For body massage the essential oils should form 2% of the blend. It is not practical to measure the essential oils in millilitres as 2% of essential oil in 10 ml of carrier oil would be 0.2 ml. The essential oils are therefore measured in drops. 1% of essential oils in 10 ml of carrier is 2.5 drops and 2% in 10 ml of carrier is 5 drops. So if you divide the millilitres of carrier oil by two the answer gives you the number of drops of essential oils to give a 2% solution, i.e. up to 5 drops of essential oils can be added to 10 ml of carrier, up to 7 drops in 14 ml and up to 10 drops in 20 ml.

For facial massage the essential oils should form 1% of the blend, half the strength of that used for the body.

The scalp can be treated with a 2% or 1% blend, whichever is the most convenient, and will need at least 5 ml of carrier oil as the hair tends to absorb some.

The oils selected for use are always the result of a careful consultation process which will take into account client preference. One, two or three essential oils may be used to make up a blend.

Factors to be considered in making up a blend

- Appropriate choice of essential and carrier oils for condition of client.
- Fragrance of individual oils acceptable to client.
- Fragrance of mix of oils acceptable to client.
- Oils with very strong fragrance used in small amounts so that they do not dominate, e.g. eucalyptus.
- Oils that complement each other.

The selection and blending of oils for use with a particular client is the most important part of the aromatherapy treatment. Some oils blend together well and are said to be acting synergically as they seem to help each other's effects. Other oils may inhibit each other's effects and do not blend so well together. If a start is made by using the oils that the client is attracted to and which fit into the category that will help the main problems the client presents, then that is an excellent start.

Examples of oils that work well together are given in the lists of essential oils.

An example of selecting a blend may be for a client who has worries at work and gets constant cold like symptoms:

- Select the general categories that suit the problems, i.e. an ester for the cooling, soothing qualities, an oxide to help the cold symptoms and maybe a ketone to loosen mucus if the cold is a chesty one.

• From the available oils, choose the ones that the client likes and that you think will go well together, e.g. lavender, eucalyptus and rosemary.

Experience will lead you to an instinctive blend of oils.

Consultation

ACTIVITY   Re-read Chapter 3 on consultation procedures.

The consultation process is especially important in clients attending for aromatherapy massage. This is because the effects of massage and the effects of the essential oils have to be considered.

The purpose of the consultation is to find out firstly that it is safe to treat the client and secondly how best to help the client.

Consultation should take into account:

1 The medical background; contra-indications, problem areas.
2 Lifestyle.
3 Personality; temperament, emotional state.

The consultation procedure to establish the medical background is fully covered in Chapter 3.

REMEMBER

You are looking for contra-indications to specific oils as well as to the massage itself.

Lifestyle and personality

Information about lifestyle and personality helps to give an overall picture of the person and indicates how you may best help them. Questions should not be too direct or probing but should be open questions allowing the client to express themselves fully.

Examples of open questions are:

• What do you feel the problem is?
• How do you think aromatherapy can help you?
• What makes you feel good/bad?

Most questions beginning with 'how', 'why', 'where', 'what', 'when' will be open questions that will give the client the opportunity to talk. Any question that can elicit the answer yes or no is a closed question. Listen to what the client wants and how they perceive their problem.

REMEMBER

Consultation is an ongoing process which should continue throughout treatment.

One useful way of asking how a client feels emotionally is to ask them to consider how they feel on a scale of 1–10 on a bad day, a good day and at the present time.

Any counselling skills that you can acquire will be of real use here in dealing with clients who have problems.

PROGRESS CHECK   With a colleague acting as a client, carry out a consultation with the aim of selecting suitable oils for the client. Ask the colleague to explain how effective the questions were in eliciting relevant information.

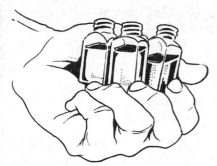

Figure 8.4 *Letting the client smell the selection*

Treatment plan following full consultation

- Decide on the aims of treatment, focusing on the client's main and secondary problems.
- List the essential oils suitable for use with these problems.
- Select two or three compatible oils from this list.
- Ask the client to smell and approve each individual oil.
- Ask the client to smell and approve the oils together.

Decide treatment method:

- Full body massage.
- Full body massage with facial massage.
- Part body massage.

Agree time scale and charges with client

Many clients may feel uncomfortable if the therapist assumes that there will be a series of treatments. Always ask if a client wants to book a series or individual treatments.

Once the treatment method and time scale have been decided the treatment plan is carried out.

Complementary home care advice should be given with the opportunity to purchase aromatherapy products. Advice might include the use of a bath oil that will complement the treatment or the use of an aromatic burner with appropriate oils.

Example

Following full consultation with a middle-aged, female client you decide the aims of treatment are:

1 General relaxation (very busy, tense lifestyle).
2 Improve sluggish circulation (cold hands and feet).

Time scale

- Ideally over a period of six weeks.
- Full body aromatherapy massage every other week alternating with an aromatherapy facial treatment.

Costs as per listed charges.

Suitable oils to use for relaxation are:

- Lavender.
- Rose geranium.
- Bergamot.

Suitable oils to use to stimulate the circulation are:

- Rosemary.
- Juniper.
- Black pepper.

Ask the client to smell each oil briefly and reject any not liked.

— REMEMBER —

Bergamot must not be used on skin to be exposed to natural or artificial sunlight.

Select two oils the client has approved, one from each group, say lavender and rosemary, and let client smell them together. If the combination is approved by the client the oils can be mixed.

- For the full body massage, in 15 ml carrier oil mix five drops of lavender and two of rosemary.
- For the facial massage, in 6 ml of carrier oil mix two drops of lavender and one of rosemary.

More than two essential oils can be used but not more than four. If three oils are preferred for the body massage the blend may be; four drops lavender, two drops rosemary, one drop bergamot.

Offer to mix oils or products for home use or take the opportunity to sell aromatherapy products. When the client returns for the next treatment always discuss the effects of the previous treatment and be ready to adjust the oils and method of application to suit the client's needs.

ACTIVITY

Keep a record of the blends you use, the clients they were used on and the results of the treatment.

Other useful essential oils

Less common essential oils are listed here in alphabetical order along with their Latin names, predominant chemical category and the effects they are best known for.

Aniseed (*Pimpinella anisum*) – middle note, ester.
- Warming, antiseptic, expectorant.

SAFE PRACTICE ▷ • *Avoid using on sensitive skin, especially allergic or inflamed skin.*

Benzoin (*Styrax benzoin*) – base note, ester.
- Anti-inflammatory, warming, good for joint conditions, colds and the skin.
- Blends well with sandalwood.

Cypress (*Cupressus sempervirens*) – middle to base note, terpene.
- Anti-rheumatic, vasoconstrictor, diuretic.
- Blends well with juniper, lavender, pine.

Fennel (*Feniculum vulgare*) – middle note, ether.
- Eases wind and stomach upsets, traditionally used for obesity.
- Blends well with geranium, lavender, sandalwood.

Immortelle (*Helichrysum angustifolium*) – middle note, ketone.

* Expectorant, good for aches and pains, skin conditions and breaks in the skin.
* Blends well with chamomile, clary sage, geranium and lavender.

Mandarin (*Citrus reticulata*) – top note, ether.

* Antiseptic, sedative.
* Blends well with other citrus oils such as neroli.

Marjoram (*Origanum majorana*) – middle note, alcohol.

* Warming, sedative, soothing, good for joint conditions.
* Blends well with lavender, rosemary, cypress and eucalyptus.

SAFE PRACTICE ▷ * *Not to be used during pregnancy.*

Myrrh (*Commiphora myrrha*) – base note, sesquiterpene.

* Healing, good for the chest, sedative.
* Blends well with frankincense, sandalwood, benzoin, juniper.

SAFE PRACTICE ▷ * *Not to be used during pregnancy.*

Myrtle (*Myrtis communis*) – middle note, oxide.

* Good for catarrh, slightly sedative, soothing.
* Blends well with bergamot, lavender, rosemary and clary sage.

Neroli or orange blossom (*Citrus aurantium*) – base note, alcohol.

* Calming, anti-stress, good for shock and depression.
* Blends well with most oils.

Patchouli (*Pogostemon cablin*) – base note, sesquialcohol.

* Good for depression, anxiety, healing skin.
* Blends well with vetiver, sandalwood, geranium, neroli.

Pine (*Pinus sylvestris*) – middle note, terpene.

* Good for colds and chest infections, stimulating.
* Blends well with tea tree, rosemary, lavender, juniper.

SAFE PRACTICE ▷ * *Avoid in cases of allergic skin condition.*

Vetiver (*Vetiveria zizanoides*) – middle note, sesquialcohol.

* Calming, stimulates the circulatory system.
* Blends well with sandalwood, patchouli, lavender and clary sage.

161

PROGRESS CHECK

1 What is an essential oil?

2 Give five factors governing the quality of an essential oil.

3 Select pairs of oils that would be suitable for use with clients who:
   a have a very stressed lifestyle
   b have problems sleeping
   c have weight and cellulite problems
   d tend to get stiff and sore after an activity such as gardening.

KEY TERMS

You need to know what these words mean. Go back through the chapter or check in the glossary to find out.

Volatile	Top note	Antiseptic
Expression	Middle note	Sedative
Distillation	Base note	Anti-oxidant
Solvent	Anti-inflammatory	Synergy

9 Aromatherapy massage and other uses for essential oils

After working through this chapter you will be able to:
- ➤ prepare a client for aromatherapy massage
- ➤ adapt the principles of body massage to aromatherapy massage
- ➤ outline the basic principles of shiatsu pressures
- ➤ apply these principles to body massage
- ➤ apply these principles to face and scalp massage
- ➤ apply these principles to massage of selected parts of the body
- ➤ give home advice to clients following aromatherapy massage
- ➤ describe other therapeutic ways of using essential oils
- ➤ recognise how aromatherapy is being used in medical settings.

Although essential oils can be used in many ways, massage is the most important and commonly used method of applying them in aromatherapy. This is because massage combines the therapeutic power of touch with the properties of the oils. Massage provides a very effective way of introducing the oils into the body. As the skin absorbs the oils, a useful amount will be taken into the bloodstream in the relatively short time that a body massage takes.

In general the conditions and legislation that cover the practice of aromatherapy will be the same as those covering the practice of massage and are described in Chapter 1.

The effects of aromatherapy massage will consist of:
- ● the effects of the massage
- ● the effects of the oils used.

Aromatherapy oils can be administered to the body using a typical body massage routine and different aromatherapists will have quite different techniques depending on their training and experience. However, in general the massage used in aromatherapy treatments is a relaxing massage using mainly effleurage and stroking movements and omitting the percussion and more vigorous petrissage movements. Instead of these more vigorous movements many therapists integrate finger pressures into their massage which may be called acupressure, shiatsu pressures or neuro-muscular techniques.

CONTRA-INDICATIONS to aromatherapy massage will consist of:

- **!** contra-indications to massage
- **!** contra-indications to the oils to be used
- **!** contra-indications to acupressure.

Acupressure

Acupressure refers to many treatment systems that manipulate the acupuncture points on the body by pressure rather than by needles as is the case with acupuncture. The acu points are found along twelve pairs of meridians or channels which pass down the body. It is said that energies flow along these meridians which govern the body's systems.

When pressure is applied to a point on a meridian it stimulates local nerves and tissues and also influences the flow of energy through that and other meridians. The basic philosophy of acu points comes from traditional Chinese systems of healing, however most Eastern societies will have pressures in their massage therapies.

Shiatsu

The Japanese word shiatsu (shi – finger, atsu – pressure) describes pressures on the acu points which may be applied with the fingers, other

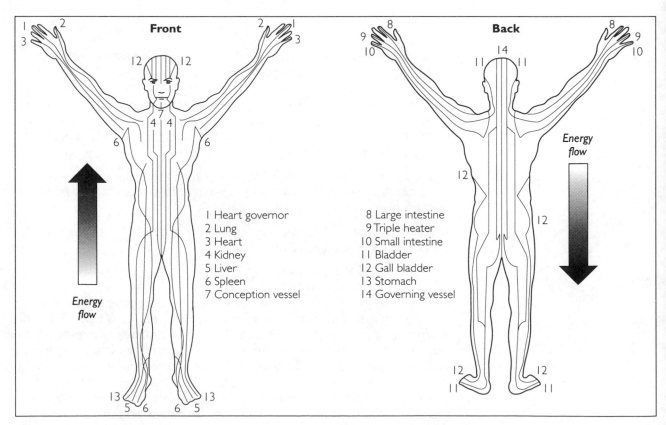

1 Heart governor
2 Lung
3 Heart
4 Kidney
5 Liver
6 Spleen
7 Conception vessel

8 Large intestine
9 Triple heater
10 Small intestine
11 Bladder
12 Gall bladder
13 Stomach
14 Governing vessel

Figure 9.1 *The meridian system*

parts of the hand and even the elbows or feet. The massage itself is just one part of a whole philosophy of treatment attempting to return the energy, or chi, of the body to a state where yin (negative) and yang (positive) qualities are in balance.

A shiatsu treatment is very different from the usual Swedish-style massage. No oil is used and there are no smooth, flowing strokes; just pressure and stretching are used. However some shiatsu-type pressures applied with the fingers or the thumb can be integrated into a Western-style massage very successfully and more can be used as a knowledge of the meridian lines is gained. Sliding pressures applied with the thumb or the hand along meridians are particularly useful as oil is being used.

Pressures

The thumbs are the usual tools used for applying pressures as the acu points are mostly placed in thumb-sized hollows. In some areas a finger may be used, often supported by the adjacent finger. The heel of the hand may be used over larger areas such as the side of the buttocks.

Pressure should be applied in a firm, controlled manner with body weight controlling the amount of pressure. No poking or roughness should be used and pressure should be moderate to light. When sliding pressure is applied it should be even and the sliding movement steady with care being taken not to cause discomfort by pulling on hair or skin.

The client should breath out when pressure is applied to the back or chest and breath in between pressures.

Pressures are usually performed only once over the area whereas the traditional massage movements will be repeated a number of times depending on the time available and the speed of the strokes.

REMEMBER

Use your hands and eyes to check the client's responses.

SAFE PRACTICE ▷ *Contra-indications to pressures are the same as those for massage, don't press over any tender or fragile areas and if pain occurs, use very light pressure. Take care that nails do not dig in.*

Routine for an aromatherapy treatment

* Consultation – which should take at least half an hour in the first instance.
* Complete consultation card.
* Obtain client's signature.
* Check for contra-indications to massage and oils.
* Select appropriate oils and check acceptability with client.
* Mix oils and check acceptability with client – mix enough 2% mixture for the body and 1% mixture for the face.
* Check that all necessary oils, creams, towels, cotton wool and tissues are close to hand.
* Suggest client empties the bladder.

REMEMBER

During treatment only the part to be worked on should be uncovered.

* An infra-red treatment may be given to warm the client, but saunas and steam baths are not suitable.
* Client lying supine, warm and well covered by towels.
* Cover the hair with a light, loose cloth or towel unless the scalp is to be included.
* If the scalp is to be included ask the client if oil may be used on the hair.
* Deep cleanse the face if facial massage is to be included.
* Place a little of the 1% oil mixture on the client's hands and ask them to inhale and lightly stroke the cheeks with the oil mixture. If there is only 2% mixture available apply a little to the client's upper lip.

SAFE PRACTICE ⊳ *Always take care to avoid getting oils in the eyes or on the eyelids.*

The order and timing of massage for an aromatherapy treatment can be adapted from the usual full body massage routine found in Chapter 6.

Suggested order and approximate timing for a full body aromatherapy massage including face and scalp

Total time taken one and a half hours.

Client turns to lie prone with hands under forehead or by sides.

1 Back, this presents the largest area for the oils to absorbed quickly – 20 minutes.
2 Back of left leg and buttock – 5 minutes.
3 Back of right leg and buttock – 5 minutes.

Client turns over to lie on back (with a pillow under the head if necessary).

4 Front of left leg and foot – 10 minutes.
5 Front of right leg and foot – 10 minutes.
6 Abdomen – 5 minutes.
7 Right arm – 5 minutes.
8 Left arm – 5 minutes.
9 Scalp – 5 minutes.
10 Face and shoulders – 20 minutes.

The routine can be adapted to suit the client and therapist. In this routine the back is treated first to allow for maximum absorption of the oils, but equally the face and scalp could be treated first.

Back

Suggested routine for back

Expose the whole length of the back from shoulders to buttocks. (Only those movements not described in Chapter 6 are explained in detail.)

1 Full back stretch (once only)

Stance   Walk or stride-standing facing across the client.

Hands   With arms straight at the elbow, one hand on upper back, other on upper part of the sacrum with the arms crossed. Apply stretch to the whole length of the spine taking care not to press the face down into the bed.

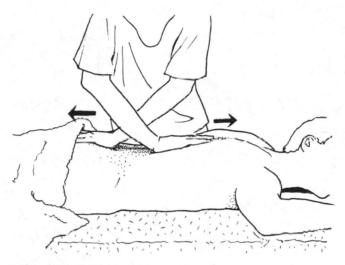

Figure 9.2   Full back stretch

2 Pressures to base of skull (once only)

Stance   Walk-standing facing the head.

Hands   One supporting head while pressure applied with the other.

Support the head with the left hand, apply pressures with right thumb on the left side of the head against the base of the skull from the outside to the centre finishing with a pressure at the centre. Repeat pressures with middle finger of right hand on the right side of the head.

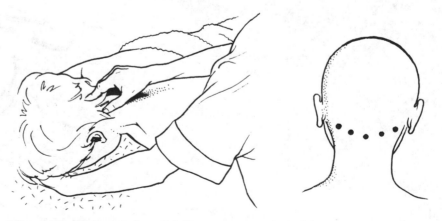

Figure 9.3   Pressures to base of skull

167

3 Apply oil to the back

Take about a third of the total oil mixed for a body massage and apply to the back with sweeping effleurage movements.

4 Reverse effleurage

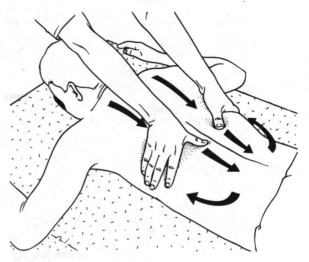

Figure 9.4   *Reverse effleurage*

5 T-shaped effleurage

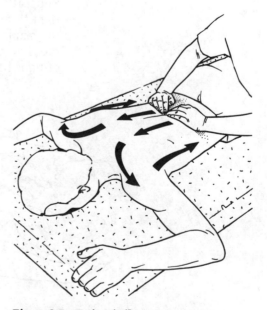

Figure 9.5   *T-shaped effleurage*

6 Circular stroking around scapulae

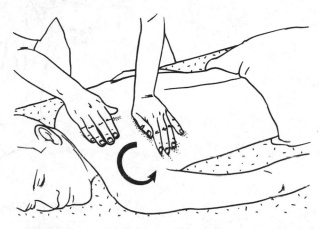

Figure 9.6 *Circular stroking around scapulae*

7 Figure of eight around scapulae

8 Pressures down side of spine (*once only*)

Stance Walk or stride-standing facing across the client.

Hands With fingertips resting lightly on the back at shoulder level, place the thumbs together and facing each other. The thumbs should be in the hollow between the spine and the erector spinae muscles of the back. Press down firmly but gently asking the client to breathe out as you press. Maintain the pressure for a count of about 4 to 5 (this can be quicker if the client requires stimulating rather than relaxation) and release, moving down a little way while the client breathes in. Pressures are applied in this way all the way down one side of the spine. The thumbs should fall naturally into the hollows between vertebrae.

9 Sliding pressures down the same side (*once only*)

Stance As for movement 8.

Hands In same position as for movement 8.

Apply steady pressure with both thumbs and keeping the pressure constant throughout, slide the lower thumb down an inch (2.5 cm) and push the other to meet it. When the level of the sacrum is reached lift the thumbs and slide the fingers up to shoulder level to repeat pressures and sliding on the other side.

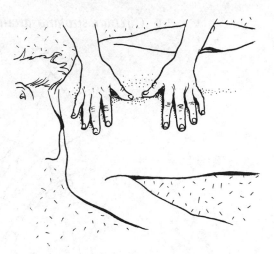

Figure 9.7 *Sliding pressures down side of spine*

10 **Pressures down other side of spine (once only)**

11 **Sliding pressures down other side of spine (once only**

12 **Wringing to the sides of the back**

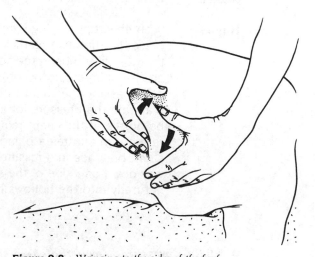

Figure 9.8 *Wringing to the sides of the back*

13 Skin rolling to sides of back

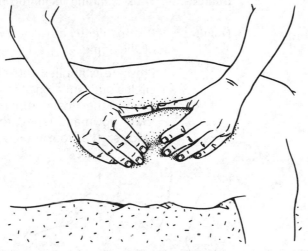

Figure 9.9   *Skin rolling to the sides of the back*

14 Effleurage towards lymph nodes (lower cervical, axillary and inguinal)

15 Transverse stroking to the lumbar region

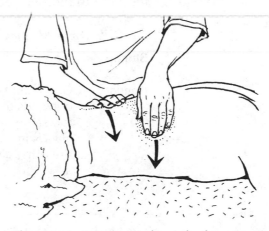

Figure 9.10   *Transverse stroking to lumbar region*

16 *Circular thumb kneading over the sacrum and iliac region*

Stance Walk-standing facing up the body.

Hands Resting lightly at waist level with the thumbs on either side of the spine.

Pressure is applied with the thumbs which move in small circles outward along the top of the iliac crest and down the sides of the hips. Return thumbs to the centre about an inch lower down and repeat the circular movements. Repeat twice so that four rows of kneadings are completed.

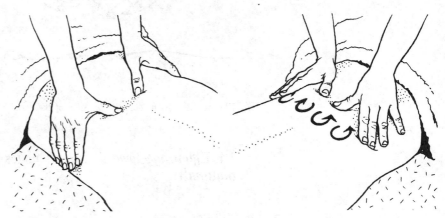

Figure 9.11 *Circular thumb kneading over the sacrum and iliac region*

Complete this movement by applying pressure with the fingers or heel of the hand to the sides of the buttocks, hold for a moment then release.

17 *Effleurage to sides of the back with alternate hands*

Stance Walk-standing facing up the body.

Hands One hand starting at base of spine, pushing upwards and outwards to the side of the body. The other hand then starts the same movement a little higher up so that one hand is always in contact until the whole side is covered. Repeat on the other side.

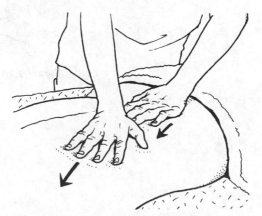

Figure 9.12 *Effleurage to side of the back with alternate hands*

18 T-shaped effleurage

Cover back with towels, tucking them in over the shoulders.

PROGRESS CHECK	**Practise this back routine until it can be performed fluently in 20 minutes.**

Legs

About a third of the remaining body oil should be used for the backs of both legs

Suggested routine for the back of the leg

(Only those movements not described in Chapter 6 are explained in detail.)

1 Apply oil to the backs of the legs

Apply oil with effleurage to whole length of both legs including feet and buttocks and cover the leg not being treated first.

2 Flat-handed effleurage with alternate hands to length of leg

Stance Stride-standing facing across the client.

Hands One hand at ankle level the other at knee level, both placed on the leg with the hands firmly cupped over the leg so that pressure is applied through the palms. not the fingers.

Move both hands slowly and steadily up the leg keeping the same distance between them and the pressure firm and steady. When the lower hand reaches the knee it is removed, but not before the upper hand reaches the top of the thigh and is brought down to ankle level. This hand now moves firmly up as far as the knee and then the free hand starts at the ankle again and they both continue together. Repeat this a number of times always with one or both hands in contact.

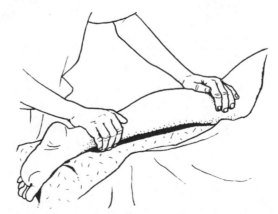

Figure 9.13 *Flat-handed effleurage with alternate hands to length of leg*

3 Wringing to thigh and buttock

4 Effleurage to thigh and buttock

5 Sliding pressure to midline of thigh with alternate hands

Stance   Walk-standing facing up the body.

Hands   One hand resting on midline of the thigh just above the knee with fingers pointing up the thigh.

Applying firm and quite deep pressure, slide the hand slowly up the thigh to the base of the buttock. Before lifting it off, start the same movement with the other hand.

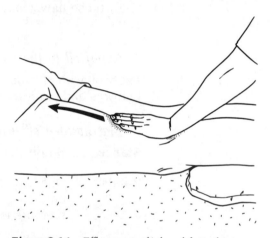

Figure 9.14   *Effleurage to thigh and buttock*

6 Effleurage to the whole leg

7 Single-handed effleurage to the calf with the knee bent

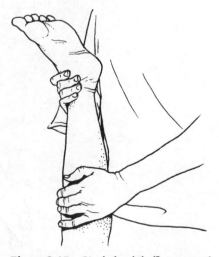

Figure 9.15   *Single-handed effleurage to the calf with the knee bent*

Stance   Walk-standing at ankle level facing up the couch.

Hands   With one hand under the ankle, lift the lower leg so that the knee is bent almost to right angles. Place the other hand so that it is cupped over the calf just above the ankle and applying pressure with the palm, stroke firmly down to the knee. Repeat a number of times and place the lower leg down gently.

8 Sliding pressures with thumbs from ankle to knee

Stance   Stand at the end of the couch.

Hands   Cupping the sides of the ankle with thumbs lying close and parallel on top of the leg

Keeping thumb tips together and applying pressure evenly with the length of the thumbs and the palms of the hands, slide the hands up to the knee. Release the pressure to return the hands to ankle level to repeat. This movement should leave a 'stocking seam' line in the oil.

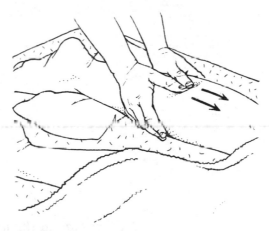

Figure 9.16   *Sliding pressures with thumbs from ankle to knee*

9 Effleurage to the whole leg.

Repeat movements 1–9 on the other leg. Ask the client to turn over and place pillows for support where necessary.

Suggested routine for front of leg

(Only those movements not described in Chapter 6 are explained in detail.)

Spread the oil with firm sweeping effleurage to both legs, including the feet, using about one third of the remaining oil.

Cover one leg with a towel.

1 Effleurage to the sides and front of the whole leg

2 *Effleurage to the thigh*

3 *Double-handed kneading to the thigh*

4 *Wringing to the thigh muscles*

5 *Stroking around the knee*

6 *Effleurage to foot and lower leg*

Stance   Walk-standing at end of couch.

Hands   One on top of and one under the foot.

Effleurage up the sides of the calf to the knee, returning with the pads of the thumbs applying gentle pressure to the tibialis muscle at the front of the leg.

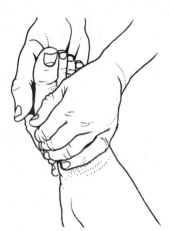

Figure 9.17   *Effleurage to foot*

7 *Effleurage to the foot*

8 *Kneading to the sole of the foot*

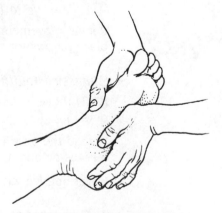

Figure 9.18   *Kneading to sole of foot*

9 Thumb stroking to the top of the foot

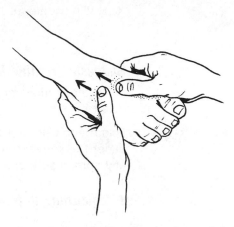

Figure 9.19   Thumb stroking to the top of the foot

10 Thumb stroking across the sole of the foot

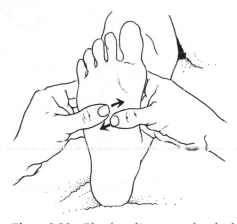

Figure 9.20   Thumb stroking across the sole of the foot

11 Kneading to the toes

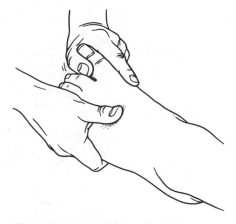

Figure 9.21   Kneading to the toes

12 *Repeat effleurage to the whole leg*

Repeat movements 1–12 on other leg.

Abdomen

Suggested routine for the abdomen

(Only those movements not described in Chapter 6 are explained in detail.)

Fold the towels back to expose the abdomen. Place small rolled-up towel under the knees to relax the abdomen. Take a third of the remaining oil and spread with clockwise circular strokes.

1 *Effleurage to front and sides of abdomen*

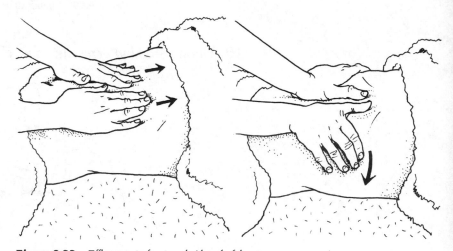

Figure 9.22 *Effleurage to front and sides of abdomen*

2 *Circular stroking in clockwise direction with alternate hands*

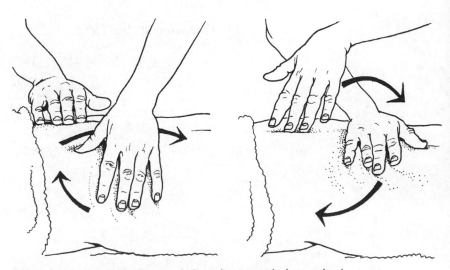

Figure 9.23 *Circular stroking in clockwise direction with alternate hands*

3 Circular kneading over the colon

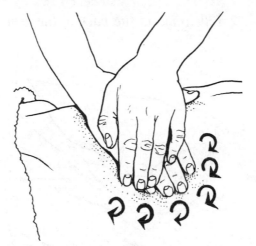

Figure 9.24   Circular kneading over colon

4 Stroking to sides of waist with alternate hands

Stance   Walk-standing at waist level facing up the couch.

Hands   One hand placed on the lower ribs strokes downward and in to the centre followed by the other hand a little lower down. Use alternate hands to cover the side from ribs to hips. Repeat on the other side

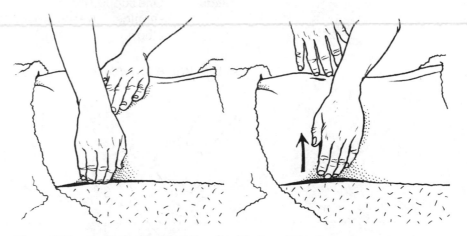

Figure 9.25   Stroking to the sides of the waist with alternate hands

5 Effleurage to front and sides of abdomen.

Arms

Suggested routine for the arms

Apply the remaining body oil to both arms using sweeping effleurage strokes. Support the arm fully during the massage.

179

1 *Effleurage to the front of the arm*

2 *Effleurage to the back of the arm including the shoulder*

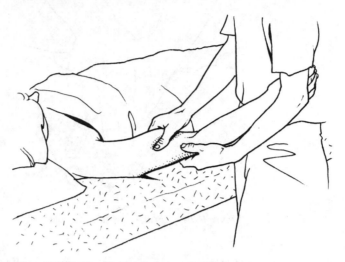

Figure 9.26 *Supporting the arm*

3 *Effleurage elbow to shoulder*

Stance   Walk-standing at waist level. The client places a hand on the chest with elbow at right angles.

Hands   One supporting the arm, the other effleurages from elbow to shoulder, sweeps around the shoulder and down to the elbow.

4 *Effleurage to forearm*

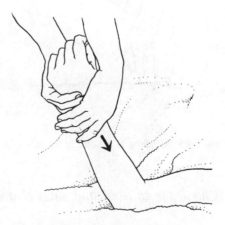

Figure 9.27 *Effleurage to the forearm*

5 Sliding pressure up midline of forearm

Stance   Walk-standing facing along the arm which should be supported.

Hands   One supporting the arm, the other resting at the front of the wrist with fingers pointing to the elbow.

Slide the hand with firm pressure up the centre of the forearm to the elbow and lightly return.

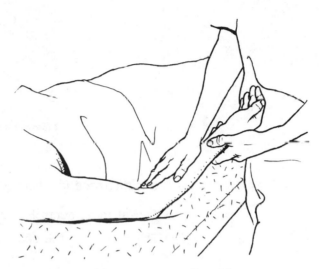

Figure 9.28   *Sliding pressure up midline of forearm*

6 Thumb stroking to the palm of the hand

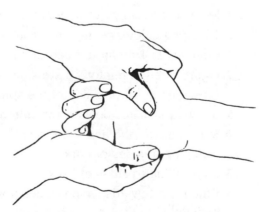

Figure 9.29   *Thumb stroking to palm of hand*

7 Thumb stroking to the back of the hand

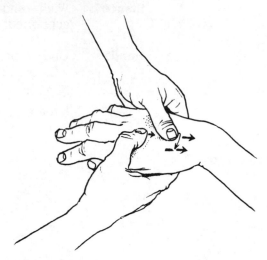

Figure 9.30 *Thumb stroking to the back of the hand*

8 Effleurage to whole arm

Repeat movements 1–8 on the other arm.

This concludes the body massage.

Summary of movements

Back

1 Full back stretch.
2 Pressures to base of skull.
3 Apply oil to whole surface of back – about a third of the total body oil can be used.
4 Reverse effleurage, shoulders to hips.
5 T-shaped effleurage, hips to shoulders.
6 Circular stroking around left and right scapulae.
7 Figure of eight reinforced stroking around the scapulae.
8 Pressures down one side of the spine.
9 Sliding pressures down same side of the spine.
10 & 11 Repeat of 8 and 9 on the other side of the spine.
12 Wringing to sides of back.
13 Skin rolling to sides of back.
14 Effleurage towards lymph nodes (lower cervical, axillary and inguinal).
15 Transverse stroking to the lumbar region.
16 Circular thumb kneading over sacrum and iliac region.
17 Effleurage to sides of back with alternate hands.
18 T-shaped effleurage.

Back of leg

1 Apply the oil with sweeping effleurage strokes to include the foot and buttock.
2 Flat-handed effleurage with alternate hands to whole leg.
3 Wringing to thigh and buttock.
4 Effleurage to thigh and buttock.
5 Sliding pressure to midline of thigh with alternate hands.
6 Effleurage to whole leg.
7 Single-handed effleurage to calf with knee bent.
8 Sliding pressures with thumbs from ankle to knee.
9 Effleurage to whole leg.

Front of leg

1 Effleurage to the sides and front of the whole leg including the foot.
2 Effleurage to the thigh.
3 Double-handed kneading to the thigh.
4 Wringing to the thigh muscles.
5 Stroking around knee.
6 Effleurage to foot and lower leg.
7 Effleurage to the foot.
8 Kneading to the sole of the foot.
9 Thumb stroking to top of foot.
10 Thumb stroking across the sole of the foot.
11 Kneading to the toes.
12 Effleurage to the whole leg.

Abdomen

1 Effleurage to front and sides of abdomen.
2 Circular stroking in clockwise direction with alternate hands.
3 Circular kneading over the colon.
4 Stroking to sides of waist with alternate hands.
5 Effleurage to front and sides of abdomen.

Arm

1 Effleurage to front of arm.
2 Effleurage to back of arm.
3 Effleurage elbow to shoulder.
4 Effleurage to forearm.
5 Sliding pressure up midline of forearm.
6 Thumb stroking to palm of hand.
7 Thumb stroking to back of hand.
8 Effleurage to whole hand.

Once the whole body massage is complete, cover the client, check for comfort and warmth and proceed with the facial and scalp massage using the 1% mixture for the face.

Facial and scalp massage

If the scalp as well as the face and chest is to be treated, then approximately 10 ml of carrier oil with 2–3 drops of essential oils will be needed. 5 ml will be adequate if only the face and chest are to be treated.

If the client prefers, the scalp can be massaged with dry hands followed by the facial massage with aromatherapy oils.

The therapist can sit at the head of the couch for part of this massage.

Scalp massage

Place a little oil in the palm of one hand and dabble the finger tips of the other in it.

1 Apply oil to the scalp

Apply the oil to the scalp with the fingertips, using small circular movements to cover the whole scalp.

2 Pressures to midline

With one thumb resting on the other, apply pressure at midline of the hairline. Release the pressure and repeat, gradually moving backwards to the crown of the head.

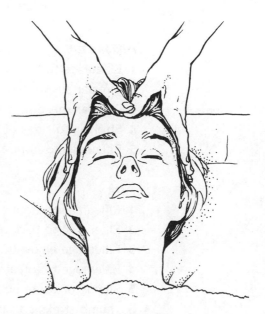

Figure 9.31 *Pressures to midline*

3 Repeat of pressures

Repeat the pressures described in movement 2 a half inch to either side of the centre with thumbs from hairline to crown and continue working outwards to temples.

4 Friction to the scalp

With fingertips clawed along the hairline, move them in deep, slow, circular movements so that the scalp moves over the bone. Gradually work backwards, altering the position of the hands so that the whole head is covered.

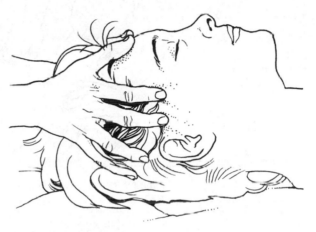

Figure 9.32 *Friction to the scalp*

5 Stroke the fingertips through the hair from hairline to ends of hair

Face

Any appropriate facial massage routine may be used so long as the neck and chest are included.

GOOD PRACTICE ▷ *The therapist should wash or wipe the hands before beginning to treat the face.*

Suggested facial routine

1 Apply oil to the face

Apply the oil with circular movements over the whole face and neck. Start with the neck, chest, shoulders, cheeks, sides of nose and forehead. Avoid the eyelids with aromatherapy oils. Finish with gentle pressure applied with the palms of the hands to both temples.

2 Effleurage to chest, shoulders and neck

Stance   Standing at the head of the couch.

Hands   Lying flat on the chest, hands pass out to the shoulders, around the points of the shoulders and up the back of the neck with a slight pull on the base of the skull.

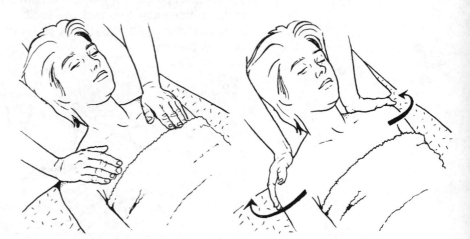

Figure 9.33   *Effleurage to chest, shoulders and neck*

3 Finger kneading to upper back

Hands   Fingers under the shoulder. Kneading to the trapezius muscles.

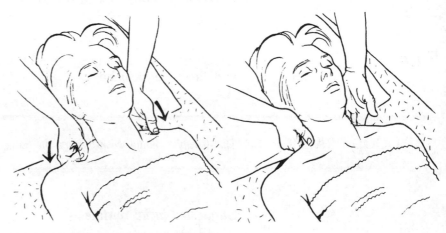

Figure 9.34   *Finger kneading to upper back*

186

4 *Effleurage to neck*

Hands   Alternate hands stroking upwards on neck from shoulders and chest to jawline to cover whole neck.

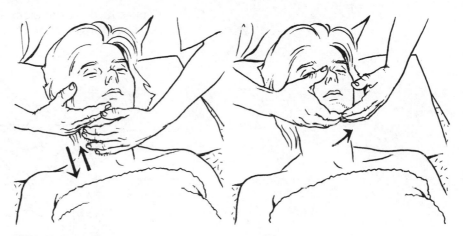

Figure 9.35   *Effleurage to neck*

5 *Effleurage chin to cheek*

Hands   Fingers linked under chin, stroke upwards to cheeks

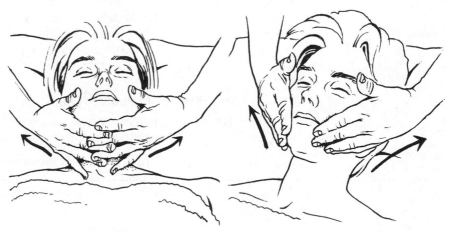

Figure 9.36   *Effleurage chin to cheek*

6 Finger pressures on cheek bones

Hands   Place thumbs on forehead and index and middle fingers on the sides of the nose. Apply pressures with the fingers along the top of the cheekbone to the temples.

Repeat lower down along the cheekbones and again along the lower edge of the cheekbones.

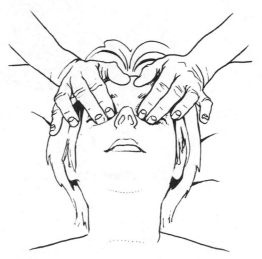

Figure 9.37   *Finger pressures on cheek bones*

7 Circular finger stroking

Hands   With middle fingers starting at the sides of the nostril, stroke up the sides of the nose to the bridge of the nose, along the top of the eyebrows down to the cheekbone and in to the sides of the nostrils again. Both fingers should move at the same time.

8 Pressures to eyebrows and forehead

Hands   Fingers resting on the temples and thumbs together between eyebrows.

Apply pressures along the length of the eyebrows then repeat an inch higher and then an inch higher again until the whole forehead is covered.

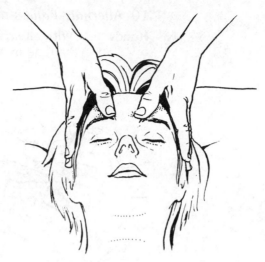

Figure 9.38 *Pressures to eyebrows*

9 *Stroking across forehead*

Hands With fingers resting on the temples and the base of the thumbs resting on the centre of the forehead, stroke outwards with the thumbs to meet the fingers.

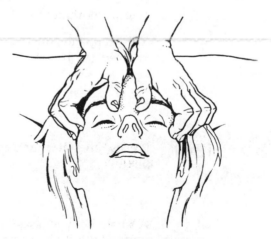

Figure 9.39 *Stroking across forehead*

10 *Alternate hand stroking to forehead*

Hands   With alternate palms, stroke upwards from temple to hairline moving across the forehead to the other temple.

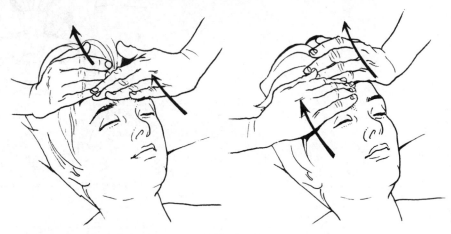

Figure 9.40   *Alternate hand stroking to forehead*

11 *Effleurage chin to cheek*

Repeat movement 5.

12 *Effleurage to chest, shoulders and neck*

Repeat movement 2.

This completes the treatment and after allowing a little time, the head of the bed can be raised to allow the client to get up.

PROGRESS CHECK   Practise the facial and scalp routine until you are able to perform it fluently

---

A whole body massage may not be required or appropriate. Individual parts of the body may be treated by aromatherapy massage taking less time and costing a proportional amount, for example:

- back massage – 30 minutes
- feet and lower legs – 15 minutes each leg
- face and scalp – 30 minutes
- face, chest and shoulders – 30 minutes.

If only a small part of the body is to be treated the essential oils used may be used in slightly stronger concentrations. 3% to 5% mixes may be used on the body, but not the face, and only if the safety of the oil has been checked.

190

ACTIVITY

Consider what types of client would benefit most from an aromatherapy massage consisting of:

a full body

b feet and lower legs

c face and scalp

d face, chest and shoulders.

Following a body massage a client should be advised to leave the oils on the body for a few hours in order to maximise the effects. It is also wise to tell the client if the oils used could have a sedative or stimulating effect, especially if the client is driving.

Further uses for essential oils

Essential oils can be used effectively in ways other than massage. They can be used in skin care by mixing them with a bland cream or adding them to a basic facial mask, in compresses, baths and be diffused into the atmosphere.

Compresses

Compresses can be hot or cold. For a hot compress, a few drops of oil can be added to a bowl of hot water and a cloth or flannel dipped in and wrung out. This can then be placed on the affected area. They are useful to place on the back, for instance, while the rest of the body is being massaged.

A cold compress is prepared in the same way using ice cold water and is suitable for the forehead if the client has a headache.

SAFE PRACTICE ▷ *Take care that the temperature of the compress is not too hot or cold before applying it to the skin.*

Baths

Essential oils can be added directly to bath water just before getting in or can be mixed with a little carrier oil first. If added directly to the water, mix the oil well in to the water before sitting in the bath to avoid them coming into direct contact with the skin. If used with a carrier oil, be careful not to slip.

Suggested oils for the bath:

* **Relaxing** – 6 drops lavender with 4 of geranium or 7 drops chamomile with 3 of basil.
* **Colds** – 6 drops of pine with 6 of eucalyptus.
* **Aches and pains** – 4 drops of rosemary with 3 of chamomile.

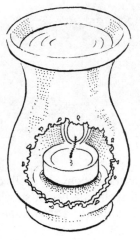

Figure 9.41 *Pottery oil burner*

Diffusion

Oils can be diffused into the atmosphere in a number of ways. The commonest way is to use a pottery burner which contains a night light candle. A few drops of oil are placed in warm water in a saucer shaped bowl above the candle. The heat from the night light speeds the evaporation of the oil into the atmosphere.

Specific oils can be chosen for their effects, e.g. frankincense and lavender for a relaxed atmosphere and eucalyptus or sweet myrtle when people have colds.

SAFE PRACTICE ▷ *Always make sure the burners cannot be accidentally knocked over.*

A more effective way of spreading oils into the atmosphere is to use an electrically operated nebulizer which propels the oil into the air in a very fine mist.

All these methods can be used to enhance and complement aromatherapy massage

Massage and aromatherapy in a medical setting

The recent growth in popularity of complementary therapies is reflected in the number of health care professionals who are showing an interest in training and in using these therapies in the treatment of patients. There is a real desire among nurses, physiotherapists and occupational therapists to return to their caring role rather than the medical model that has been the trend for many years. The term 'holistic approach' is being used more and more where all aspects of the individual being treated are considered rather than just the physical.

Some recent examples of massage and aromatherapy being used in such a way follow.

Labour ward

Midwives at the John Radcliffe Maternity Hospital in Oxford wanting to find a way of relieving pain and calming women in labour set out to evaluate the use of essential oils for the purpose. The project lasted six months and the oils used were lavender, clary sage, peppermint, eucalyptus, chamomile, frankincense, jasmine, rose, lemon and mandarin.

The oils were used in baths, footbaths, inhaled or massaged. The most effective oil used was lavender. Peppermint and clary sage also showed good results. There was a high degree of satisfaction from the women and the midwives and the use of essential oils has been retained in the labour ward.

Intensive care

Research in the intensive and coronary care unit of the Royal Sussex County Hospital showed that massage and the use of essential oils reduced the heart rate and breathing rate in most of the patients tested and seemed to be more effective than massage alone.

The feet were massaged with lavender in a carrier oil and comparison was made with patients who were massaged with carrier oil alone. The drop in the heart rate was significantly greater in the lavender group.

Occupational Therapy

Aromatherapy and massage are currently being used by many occupational therapists in a variety of settings to develop relationships, relieve anxiety and to help physical function. One example is where the occupational therapist massages the hands of children using lavender oil to relax and mobilise the hands before exercise. Other uses may be to diffuse into the atmosphere to promote concentration or relaxation.

Sleep patterns

A trial to evaluate the effects of lavender diffusion on the sleep patterns of patients with dementia was carried out in 1993 at Newholme Hospital, Bakewell. The trial ran over a seven week period using an electric diffuser. The results showed a significant improvement in the sleep patterns of the patients.

ACTIVITY

Try to carry out a literature search in professional journals and collect references to the use of massage and aromatherapy in a variety of medical settings.

KEY TERMS

You need to know what these words mean. Go back through the chapter or check in the glossary to find out.

Therapeutic	Acupressure	Diffusion
Shiatsu	Compress	

Bibliography and further reading

Barclay, J. *The Story of Care in Our Hands*. Physiotherapy, May 1994 vol. 80 no. 5.

Beck, M. *The Theory and Practice of Therapeutic Massage*. Milady Publishing Company, 1988.

Brown, Denise. *Aromatherapy*. Headway Lifeguides Series, 1993.

Burns, E., Blamey, C. *Soothing Scents in Childbirth*. The International Journal of Aromatherapy, 1994 vol. 4 no. 1.

Corbett, M. *The Use and Abuse of Massage and Exercise*. The Practitioner, Jan 1972 vol. 208.

Corney, J. *Anthropometry for Designers*. Batsford Academic and Educational Ltd. London, 1980.

Cowmeadow, O. *The Art of Shiatsu*. Element Books Ltd., 1992.

Davis, P. *Aromatherapy an A–Z*. C.W. Daniel Company Ltd., 1990.

Ernst, E. et al. *Massages Cause Changes in Blood Fluidity*. Physiotherapy, 1987 vol. 73 no. 1.

Fire, M. *Providing Massage Therapy in a Psychiatric Hospital*. International Journal of Alternative and Complementary Medicine, June 1994.

Gallant, Ann. *Body Treatments and Dietetics for the Beauty Therapist*. Stanley Thornes (Publishers) Ltd., 1978.

Gillam, L. *Lymphoedema and Physiotherapists: Control not Cure*. Physiotherapy, December 1994 vol. 80 no.12.

Goldberg, A. G. *Body Massage for the Beauty Therapist*. Heinmann, 1972.

Grisogono, V. *Sports Injuries*. Churchill Livingstone, 1989.

Henry, J. et al. *Lavender for Night Sedation of People with Dementia*. International Journal of Aromatherapy, 1994 vol. 6 no. 2.

Herring, M. *Aromatherapy – Making Connections*. The International Journal of Aromatherapy, 1994 vol. 6 no. 1.

Hollis, M. *Massage for Therapists*. Blackwell Scientific Publications, 1987.

Hotchkiss, S. *How thin is your skin?* New Scientist, Jan. 1994.

Hovind, H., Nielsen, S. *Effect of Massage on Blood Flow in Skeletal Muscle*. Scandinavian Journal of Rehabilitation Medicine, Med 6: 74–77, 1974.

International School of Aromatherapy. *A Safety Guide on the Use of Essential Oils*. Nature by Nature Oils Ltd. London, 1993.

Lawless, Julia. *The Encyclopaedia of Essential Oils*. Element Books Ltd. Dorset, 1992.

Lidell, L., Thomas, S., Beresford Cooke, C., Porter, A. *The Book of Massage*. Ebury Press, 1987.

Lavabre, M. *Aromatherapy Workbook*. Healing Arts Press, USA, 1990.

Marshall Cavendish. *How the Body Works*. Marshall Cavendish London, 1979.

Maxwell Hudson, C. *The Complete Book of Massage*. Dorling Kindersley Pub. Ltd., 1988.

Minett, P., Wayne, D., Rubenstein, D. *Human Form and Function*. Collins International, 1992.

Price, S. *Practical Aromatherapy*. Thorsons Publishing Group, 1987.

Quinter, J. *Apropos Rub, Rub, Rubbish; Massage in the Ninteenth Century*. Physiotherapy, 1993 vol. 79 no. 1.

Roberts, P. *Theoretical Models of Physiotherapy*. Physiotherapy, June 1994 vol. 80 no. 6.

Sanderson, H., Ruddle, J. *Aromatherapy and Occupational Therapy*. British Journal of Occupational Therapy, 1992, 55(8).

Simms, J. *A Practical Guide to Beauty Therapy*. Stanley Thornes (Publishers) Ltd., 1993.

Sigerist, H. E. *A History of Medicine*. Oxford University Press Inc., 1951.

Tisserand, R. *Aromatherapy Today*. The International Journal of Aromatherapy, 1993 vol. 5 no. 4.

Tortora, G., Anagnostakos, N. P. *Principles of Anatomy and Physiology* (3rd Ed.). Harper International.

Woolfson, A., Hewitt, D. *Intensive Aroma Care*. International Journal of Aromatherapy, 1992 vol. 4 no. 2.

Ylinen, J., Cash, M. *Sports Massage*. Stanley Paul & Co. Ltd. London, 1988.

Glossary

Adipose tissue – connective tissue containing fat cells.

Alimentary canal – the tube extending from the mouth to the anus.

Allergens – a substance which causes an allergy.

Allergy – an extreme sensitivity to certain substances or allergens.

Alveoli – air sacs in the lungs.

Antibody – a protein substance in the blood which is formed by lymphocytes to combat disease.

Antigens – a substance which stimulates the production of antibodies.

Appendicular skeleton – the bones of the limbs and the two girdles.

Arterioles – small branches of arteries which end in capillaries.

Autonomic nervous system – the part of the nervous system that regulates the internal organs, made up of the sympathetic and parasympathetic divisions. The effects of each counteracts and balances the effects of the other.

Axial skeleton – the central part of the skeleton, skull, vertebral column and bones of the trunk.

Axilla – the armpit.

Bronchioles – small tubes in the lung leading to the alveoli.

Capillary – very small blood vessels which connect the arteries and veins.

Cartilage – tough, flexible connective tissue found in parts of the body needing firm support.

Collagen – tough, inelastic material which is a constituent of connective tissue and bone.

Connective tissue – contains different types of cells and fibres, it holds other tissues and organs together and gives them support.

Contra-indication – a condition indicating that a treatment must not be carried out.

Closed question – a question that can be answered with a simple yes or no.

Dermis – the deep layer of the skin containing blood vessels, nerves, glands, hair roots and connective tissue.

Desquamation – the removal of the surface cells of the skin.

Dextrous – the skilful, precise use of the hands.

Diffusion – a method of evenly spreading fine droplets of a fluid into the air.

Distal – the furthest point of a limb from the body.

Effleurage – stroking massage movements in the direction of venous and lymphatic flow.

Endocrine glands – those glands which produce chemical messengers (hormones) which are carried in the blood stream and are responsible for maintaining homeostasis.

Enzyme – a protein substance acting as a catalyst for chemical reactions in the body.

Epidermis – the tough outer layer of the skin which protects the deeper tissues.

Erythema – a superficial redness of the skin.

Friction – a brisk rubbing of the skin to produce warmth.

Gluteal – the region over the buttocks.

Hazard – danger.

Histamine – a chemical substance released by the mast cells in the skin as a result of irritation, causing itching, redness and weals.

Holism – a concept of health which includes the whole person, physical and psychological.

Homeostasis – the maintenance of the internal environment of the body.

Hormone – the chemical messengers produced by the endocrine glands.

Hygiene – the state of cleanliness, environmental and personal.

Keratin – insoluble protein which is the main component of hair and nails.

Ligament – band of tough inelastic connective tissue joining bone to bone at joints.

Limbic system – a part of the brain closely related to the thalamus and hypothalamus thought to affect the emotions.

Lymph – a yellowish fluid contained in the lymphatic vessels. It is similar to tissue fluid but contains more protein.

Lymph nodes – often called lymph glands, they are small bean-shaped bodies situated along lymph vessels which filter the lymph and make lymphocytes and antibodies.

Lymphocytes – white blood cells which make antibodies to destroy bacteria or viruses.

Mailshot – letters sent to a large number of customers as an advertisement.

Metabolic rate – the amount of energy used by a body in a set time.

NCVQ – National Council for Vocational Qualifications.

Open questions – questions which cannot be answered with a simple yes or no.

Osteopathy – method of treatment by manipulation.

Patch test – application to a small patch of skin of a substance suspected of causing a reaction.

Patella – kneecap.

Peristalsis – the rhythmic muscular movement of the bowel which moves food onwards.

Petrissage – massage movements which involve pressing and squeezing the tissues.

pH value – acidity/alkalinity maintained at a constant level in the body.

Physiotherapy – the treatment of disease, disability or injury by physical means.

Phytohormones – hormone-like substances found in plants.

Popliteal – the area at the back of the knee.

Prone – lying face down.

Proximal – the part of a limb closest to the body.

Receptors – sensory structures receiving stimuli.

Reflex – an involuntary response to a stimulus.

Renal – relating to the kidneys.

Rolling – massage movements where the tissues are rolled between thumb and fingers.

Sedative – slows down activity.

Shiatsu – a method of physical treatment involving pressures on certain points of the body.

Stress – psychological pressure caused by situations or other people.

Supine – lying face upwards.

Synergy – working together to the benefit of each.

Synovial – relating to the synovial membrane that surrounds freely moveable joints and which produces synovial fluid.

Tapotement – massage movements that involve tapping or percussion on the body.

Tendon – tough bands of inelastic connective tissue linking muscle to bone.

Tension – the body's reaction to stress.

Therapy – any form of treatment.

Thrombus – a clot of blood in the heart or blood vessels.

Toxin – any substance which causes damage to tissues.

Traction – gentle stretching of a part, especially related to joints.

Ulnar – the little finger side of the arm or hand.

Urinary – related to the function of the bladder.

Venule – the small veins which are the termination of the venous system.

Volatile – oils that may be vaporised into the atmosphere.

Useful addresses

Equipment (couches)

Carlton Professional

Carlton House
Commerce Way
Lancing
West Sussex BN15 8TA
Tel: 01903 761100

New Concept Treatment Couches

Cox Hall Lane
Tattingstone
Ipswich
Suffolk IP9 2NS
Tel: 01473 328006

Nomeq

23/24 Thornhill Road
North Moons Moat
Redditch
Worcestershire B98 9ND
Tel: 01527 64222

Associations

Aromatherapy Organisations Council

3 Latymer Close
Braybrooke
Market Harborough
Leicestershire LE16 8LN
Tel: 01858 434242

British Association of Beauty Therapy and Cosmetology

Parabola Road
Cheltenham
Gloucestershire GL50 3AH
Tel: 01242 570284

Institute for Complementary Medicine

PO Box 194
London SE16 1QZ
Tel: 0171 237 5165

International Federation of Aromatherapists
Stamford House
2/4 Chiswick High Road
London W4 1TH
Tel: 0181 742 2605

The Register of Qualified Aromatherapists
PO Box 6941
London N8 9HF
Tel: 0181 341 2958

Journals

Health and Beauty Salon

Quadrant House
The Quadrant
Sutton
Surrey SM2 5AS
Tel: 0181 652 8268

The International Journal of Aromatherapy
Box 746
Hove
East Sussex BN3 3XA
Tel: 01273 772479

Journal of Alternative and Complementary Medicine
Green Library
Homewood NHS Trust
Guildford Road
Chertsey
Surrey KT16 OQA
Tel: 01932 872777

Oils

Saffron Oils
Belmont House
Newport
Saffron Walden
Essex CB11 3RF
Tel: 01799 540622

Shirley Price Aromatherapy Oils
Essentia House
Upper Bond Street
Hinckley
Leicestershire LE10 1RS
Tel: 01455 615 466

Tisserand Aromatherapy Products
Newtown Road
Hove
East Sussex BN3 7BA
Tel: 01273 325666

Index